ROBERT CRAYHON'S
NUTRITION
MADE SIMPLE

ROBERT CRAYHON'S
NUTRITION
MADE SIMPLE

A Comprehensive Guide to the Latest Findings in Optimal Nutrition

Robert Crayhon, M.S.

Certified Nutritionist

M. Evans and Company, Inc.
New York

M. Evans and Company, Inc.
216 East 49th Street
New York, New York 10017

Library of Congress Cataloging-in-Publication Data

Crayhon, Robert, 1961–
    Robert Crayhon's Nutrition made simple : a comprehensive guide to
the latest findings in optimal nutrition / Robert Crayhon.
       p.   cm.
    Includes bibliographical references and index.
    ISBN 0-87131-796-6
    1. Nutrition.   2. Health.   I. Title.
RA784.C65   1996
613.2–dc20   95-43216
                                                        CIP

Design by Charles A. de Kay
Typeset by AeroType, Inc.

Manufactured in the United States of America
9 8 7 6 5 4 3 2

The advice offered in this book, although based on the author's experience with many thousands of patients, is not intended to be a substitute for the advice and counsel of your personal physician.

This book is dedicated to
my mother, Ann Conroy, and
my father, Joseph Crayhon.

Acknowledgments

I WOULD LIKE TO THANK DON Brown, N.D.; Mary Enig, Ph.D.; Brian Leibovitz, Ph.D.; and Natasha Trenev for their expert advice. I would also like to thank Jane Jeffs for her many valuable suggestions; Linda Lizotte for covering for my office hours so I could write this book, and for giving me her excellent input; and Jonathan Lizotte, for his comments and input.

Contents

FOREWORD

THIS BOOK, *ROBERT CRAYHON'S NUTRITION MADE SIMPLE,* is clear, direct, and right up to the minute . . . just like Robert Crayhon himself. Robert has tackled the ever-changing, often confusing science of nutrition and made this fascinating subject user-friendly and concise. He presents a refreshing look at the most current issues of the day—ranging from nutrition basics to supplements to body health, health problems, weight loss, and preventitive medicine—in a way that does not merely rehash the same information over and over again. Robert offers both useful and innovative material in his discussion of good health that goes far beyond the current dietary wisdom so many of us take as gospel.

In the very first chapters of the book you will see how Robert forges ahead of the standard nutritional dogma by openly challenging some basic beliefs about optimum diet and health. He goes on to dismantle the notion that the popular low-fat, high-complex-carbohydrate diet is the universal panacea for every man and woman with regard to total wellness. He even goes so far as to say that one diet plan may not be right for everybody and that we would do well to consider our ancestry and heredity. Although this may seem like news to us in the 1990s, Robert's insights are well founded in research done in the earlier part of the century by brilliant nutrition pioneers. And all of this . . . just for starters.

For years I have maintained just what Robert is writing about. I have counseled thousands of individuals and written my own books to provide a nutritional point of view that takes into consideration the latest research developments and personal, everyday counseling experience. *Robert Crayhon's Nutrition Made Simple* will give many more people the opportunity to consider all facets of nutrition and not be stuck with the simplest notion that you can eat what you want, whenever you want, as long as your food is fat-free and full of fiber. Nutrition is a far more interesting and richer subject than just the association with fat, fat grams, and fat obsession.

Indeed, the reader will quickly discover how varied a subject nutrition can be. There is something for everyone in this book. Senior citizens are represented as well as specific female concerns like PMS and osteoporosis. Natural approaches to arthritis, heart disease, and even stopping smoking are explored. And for those with digestive problems and lack of energy, there are answers. The chapter on "How to Find a Good Nutritionist" should be of particular interest to every health-minded reader who is in search of a qualified practitioner.

I first met Robert several years ago when he invited me to be a guest on his radio show. I quickly became very impressed with this young man who asked all the right questions and had journal citations on a variety of topics at the tip of his tongue. I later learned that Robert has maintained a busy practice in Mamaroneck, New York, and New York City for many years. As the host of the "Voice of Wellness," a nationally syndicated health and wellness radio program, Robert is in touch with real people and their day-to-day health problems and questions. He is not just an armchair nutritionist writing a book. His knowledge comes from daily practice and observation. In fact, Robert was named one of the Top Ten Nutritionists in America by *Self* magazine in August of 1993.

Men, women, and health care practitioners (especially doctors) should read Robert's book to learn not only what they *want* to know about nutrition, but what they really *need* to know. Robert's unique sense of humor, which prevails throughout, makes his book enjoyable—almost fun reading. It seems to me that *Robert Crayhon's Nutrition Made Simple* will become a landmark guide for nutrition in the '90s. I can't wait for the sequel.

Ann Louise Gittleman, M.S.
Certified Nutrition Specialist
Bozeman, Montana

When we silence any voice, we rob ourselves of part of the truth.

—J. S. Mill, *On Liberty*

Preface

THIS IS A BOOK ABOUT optimal nutrition, not adequate nutrition. A book on adequate nutrition would be about as interesting as a financial guide for staying above the poverty level. Nutrition that merely prevents deficiencies pales compared to optimal nutrition, which can promote vibrant health and prevent degenerative disease. It is the difference between the lightning bug and lightning.

Optimal nutrition goes well beyond the RDA. It helps us understand what the most beneficial level of intake for all nutrients is, not the lowest amounts we can survive on. Correctly implemented, it has the power to decrease the incidence of heart disease, cancer, and a myriad of diseases related to the immune system. It can increase worker productivity, lower health-care costs, save marriages, increase intelligence, prevent birth deformities, and increase the quality and length of life.

Some say that nutrition is still too young a science and that optimal levels of nutrients are not yet known. While we still have much to learn, implementing what we already know would be of untold benefit. Thousands of studies have shown the powerfully preventive and therapeutic role of nutrients such as vitamins C, E, folic acid, magnesium, zinc, and selenium. The amounts found in food are not enough. We must use supplements. We have arrived at a point at which we will either use this knowledge and protect our bodies with optimal levels of nutrients or be bankrupted by health-care costs. Degenerative diseases are a luxury we can no longer afford.

Even if Americans consumed the RDA for every nutrient, they would still be far from optimally healthy. The amounts that prevent deficiency diseases do not prevent degenerative diseases. We need to abandon the RDA as a butterfly does its cocoon and realize that vibrant life comes from seeking new, optimal levels of intake for all essential nutrients.

Our culture has a schizophrenic approach to wellness. There is a Dunkin' Donuts inside the Harvard School of Public Health. In 1992 the National Cancer Institute spent $400,000 to encourage people to eat vegetables. That same year, Kellogg spent $49 million to convince children to eat sugary cereals. The government spends money to convince people not to smoke while subsidizing tobacco farmers. We may want health, but big business is sacred. The biggest of them all is crisis-care medicine.

The health-care or crisis-care system is a cancer. It depends upon a steady stream of illness to keep its engine going, and nothing threatens it more than a nation that could keep itself healthy. We don't need to get a better health-care system. We need to get rid of it and create a new one that actually prevents diseases instead of profiting from them. We aren't preventing anything in this country. Most physicians cover up symptoms with medications or remove troublesome organs with surgery. High blood pressure and cholesterol-lowering medications look preventive, but studies show they decrease lifespan.

Medicine does not need any more technological advances; it needs an intellectual revolution. It must spend less time studying how the body gets ill and expend more effort to understand the forces that keep it healthy. Hospitals have become diagnostic amusement parks and have no overall strategy for generating wellness. They only make money if you become sick enough to need crisis care. And it is in these centers for crisis-care medicine that most modern physicians are trained.

The extraordinary crisis medicine that separates Siamese twins and reattaches digits is breathtaking, but it affects very few of us. It does, however, mesmerize us into the false belief that all medicine is state of the art. Some medicine is in the Space Age. Preventive medicine is in the Stone Age. We need high-tech medicine mostly because we need to be rescued from the diseases caused by our ignorance of aggressive preventive medicine. Until there is financial reward for prevention, we can expect medicine to remain crisis care.

THE DANGERS OF NUTRITION

There are two dangers to nutrition. The first is to think too much of it. Even optimal nutrition cannot completely reverse damage to the body from disease, stress, toxins in our environment, or years of poor eating habits.

The second danger of nutrition, however, is far more perilous. It is to think too little of it. Optimal nutrition offers a powerful defense against the onslaught of degenerative diseases. It is the cornerstone of the treatment and prevention of every ailment. Optimal intake of all nutrients combined with a healthy, toxin-free diet has become a necessity in our polluted world. Only by seeking to maximize our health in all ways possible, through a positive mental outlook, exercise, and the most nutrient-dense diet possible, can we hope to lower the rates of heart disease, cancer, osteoporosis, senility, and a host of other degenerative diseases that will otherwise decrease the quality and length of all of our lives. Thanks to the science of optimal nutrition, we have information that may one day make these ailments a thing of the past.

Part I
The Basics

CHAPTER 1

What Is Health?

Everything depends upon what people are capable of wanting.
—Enrico Malatesta

HEALTH REQUIRES BALANCE

The American puritanical heritage often keeps us from understanding the nature of health. We start by classifying everything as good or bad:

Good	Bad
Starches	Fat
Exercise	Inactivity
Thinness	Obesity
Drugs	Viruses
Antibiotics	Bacteria
Vitamins and Minerals	Toxins
Antioxidants	Free Radicals
Avoiding Sunlight	Sunburn

The ideas of good and bad distract us from the most important concept of all: balance. We are trained to eradicate all that is "bad" and to get as much as possible of all that is "good." Taken to extremes, this approach to wellness does not work.

Everything Is Needed in a Balanced Amount
Copper is a mineral that is part of a protective antioxidant enzyme and keeps cholesterol, blood pressure, insulin, and blood sugar in a normal range. But in excessive amounts, copper will generate damaging free radicals. Exercise is one of the most important parts of a healthy lifestyle. Yet too much exercise will lead to adrenal exhaustion. Whole grains and

19

beans are health-promoting, but eaten to the exclusion of all other foods, can lead to low energy and poor immune function. "Fat-free" foods are sold to a nation deficient in essential fatty acids. With all of our dietary puritanism, Americans are more overweight and diseased than ever.[1] We start off with good ideas. But because we lack balance in our overall concept of wellness, we take our approach too far in one direction and use them to create illness.

Everything must be appreciated as part of a balanced whole. This is not a credo of a mystical religion; it is a scientific fact. If we fail to appreciate and employ balance in all things, we will never achieve a higher level of wellness no matter how much nutrition information we amass.

An Unhealthy Nation

If you are like most Americans, you are developing a preventable disease. Almost everyone has clogging arteries. The vast majority of Americans have a deficiency of the mineral chromium, which can lead to blood sugar instability and diabetes. A large portion of the population have magnesium and zinc deficiencies, which can cause heart and prostate disorders. Few of us receive adequate amounts of antioxidant nutrients such as vitamins C, E, and the trace mineral selenium. This increases our risk for certain types of cancer. Essential omega-3 fatty acids are also missing, creating an even wider range of problems.

All of this is accepted as perfectly normal.

We have an accepted level of illness in America. As long as you are progressing at the same rate as everyone else, you are considered healthy. Your health has more to do with your test results than the state of your body. If you have clogging arteries, decaying teeth, toxic metal contamination, exhausted adrenal glands, a liver that does not function optimally, a high body fat percentage, and low levels of many essential nutrients, you may still be called "perfectly healthy."

Our number one health problem is our definition of health. We call the absence of disease health. "If it ain't broke, don't fix it" is our credo. When people discover they have breast cancer, prostate cancer, severely clogged arteries, or bone deterioration, it wasn't something that happened that day that caused their health to suddenly deteriorate. It was the result of a life of unhealthy eating, suboptimal nutrient intake, overwork, poor stress management, and destructive habits such as smoking. But until a disease formally introduces itself, we don't want to think about it.

In America, wellness is an abnormality. *Health nut*—a derogatory term for someone who wants optimal health—shows how out of step with a disease-ridden society someone is who wants high-level wellness. Do we call millionaires wealth nuts?

We need a new standard for wellness known as *optimal health.* We need bodies that are as healthy as possible, not merely alive. Otherwise, we are just sitting ducks for whatever degenerative disease strikes first. There is no middle ground.

Ed: Case of Adequate Health

Ed doesn't drink or smoke, but he doesn't watch what he eats. His kids like fast-food restaurants, so he frequents them. His blood pressure, cholesterol, and other tests are normal. Ed takes high blood pressure medicine, which seems to be working. "You're perfectly healthy," his doctor says. He isn't. He just doesn't have acute conditions. One hopes he won't develop any. But should he, he and his doctor will do little more than try to manage them with more medications.

Tom's Goal: Optimal Health

Tom exercises regularly and has a positive self-image. He does his best to eat well, even though he eats out a lot. He supplements with nutrients that are not supplied in optimal amounts by his diet such as vitamins C, E, B complex, selenium, and chromium. He avoids toxic foods like margarine and fried foods. He consumes a lot of produce, and buys organic when he can find it. He can even be seen making fresh vegetable juice on weekends. He takes a ginkgo supplement because of its benefits on brain health. He visits regularly with a nutritionist who guides him toward the best combination of food and supplements for his metabolism. His hair analysis detected high levels of a toxic metal called cadmium. He takes extra zinc and other nutrients to help rid himself of it before it can cause disease. Tom doesn't drink coffee. He has switched to green tea for his morning caffeine. He read that it has helped the Japanese stay healthy. He also gives blood once per year to keep his iron in an optimal range and tracks his iron levels annually with a serum ferritin test.

Tom is successful at his job, but does not overwork. He has burned himself out before and now rejects projects that may not allow him adequate rest and enjoyment. He thinks in the long run it may cost him a promotion, but he would rather be happy and have more time for his family.

Tom watched his father decline into Alzheimer's disease and does not want that or a similar disease to happen to him. He doesn't eat a perfect diet, but he does his best. His habits have greatly reduced his chances of getting a degenerative disease.

The way to solve the health-care crisis is to turn the Eds of America into Toms. That requires education and personal involvement. It requires fast-food restaurants that serve healthier foods for times when Ed takes his kids out for a meal. It requires food manufacturers that make fresher, less-processed foods with shorter shelf life to help you live a longer life. A country and a food processing industry divided against themselves cannot stand.

THE PRINCIPLES OF OPTIMAL HEALTH

1. A Positive Self-Image
2. A Diet Free of Toxic Foods That Supplies Optimal Levels of All Beneficial Nutrients
3. Clean Air and Living Environment, Pure Water, and Adequate Sunshine
4. Adequate Exercise and Rest

Positive Mental Outlook

You cannot be healthy on any level until you are healthy on every level. The key to it all is a positive self-image. Until you have adequate self-esteem, all of the information you amass about getting healthy will do you no good, for you will not think highly enough of yourself to use it.

Along with self-esteem, we need to cultivate personal responsibility. No one keeps you healthy. Nutritionists, nutritionally oriented physicians, naturopaths, osteopaths, and chiropractors coach. It is up to you to keep yourself healthy.

Optimal Intake of All Beneficial Nutrients

Adequate amounts of essential nutrients will eliminate deficiencies, but will not prevent cancer or heart disease. Even a high-potency multivitamin, while a good start, is only the beginning. You need to get all forty-five nutrients in optimal amounts. These amounts will differ for each person and his or her unique metabolism and lifestyle.

We need, however, more than just the ones that are essential: We need all that are *beneficial*. We need to examine so-called nonessential nutrients such as CoQ10, carnitine, GLA, taurine, and N-Acetyl Cysteine (NAC). While these nutrients are made by the body in small amounts, the only way to get them in optimal amounts is through supplements. Other nonessential protective substances include polyphenols from plants that have tremendous protective and therapeutic ability.[2, 3] Investigate all nutrients and take those you find most helpful. All beneficial nutrients are essential for those who want health at the highest level.

Avoid Toxic Foods and Contaminants

- Margarine, vegetable shortenings, and baked goods containing "partially hydrogenated oil"
- Fried foods of all kinds, including fried chips from the health food store. Stir-frying is okay.
- Supermarket vegetable oils such as corn, sunflower, safflower, and canola oils that have had all of the nutrients refined out of them. These nutritionally naked junk oils contain toxic trans fats, are often rancid, and cause disease. Consume only virgin flax, canola, and olive oils that are stored in opaque containers and pressed at low temperatures from organic sources.
- White flour, bleached flour, bromated flour, even "wheat flour." It has to say "whole wheat flour." If it does not say "whole wheat" or "whole grain," avoid it.
- Unless you are a menstruating woman, avoid Product 19, Total, and all cereals and foods that have the full RDA for iron added to them. The overconsumption of iron poses a serious health threat for men and postmenopausal women.
- Sugar in all forms: high-fructose corn syrup, barley malt, fruit juice concentrate, honey, molasses, maple syrup, invert sugar, etc.
- Avoid baking powder that contains aluminum, aluminum foil, and aluminum pots and pans. Aluminum is implicated in causing Alzheimer's disease.
- Coffee, caffeinated or not. It is loaded with pesticides and free-radical-producing hydrocarbons, and stains your spleen and liver the color of the bottom of a coffee cup.

- Additives: Buy food that does not have chemical preservatives, artificial colors, emulsifiers, or other synthetic agents. Americans eat many pounds of these chemicals per year and have the toxic bodies to prove it.
- Foods that you may be sensitive to. Wheat, gluten-containing grains, dairy products, and yeast-containing foods are common offenders. Your nutritionist or holistic M.D. can help you pinpoint foods that may be troublesome for you.
- Produce grown with pesticides, fungicides, and herbicides. Eat vegetables no matter what kind you buy, but organic produce is best. Organic foods are those grown without harmful chemicals. Pesticides have been implicated in causing a wide range of diseases including cancer and impaired brain function in the elderly.
- Avoid peanuts and peanut butter unless the manufacturer certifies them aflatoxin-free. Aflatoxin is a powerfully carcinogenic mold that grows easily on these legumes as well as corn and is believed to cause thousands of cases of liver cancer per year.
- Chicken, meat, and eggs from animals fed hormones and antibiotics. Free-range animals have more essential fatty acids, less total fat, and make healthier meat and eggs.
- Avoid fish from polluted waters. Raw or undercooked fish should also be avoided as it can harbor parasites.
- Keep alcohol consumption to a minimum, and make organic red wine your drink of choice if you drink.

A Clean Environment

Pure water that is free of fluoride (once used as a rat poison), chlorine, and other toxins is essential to good health. Buy spring or distilled water or invest in a high-quality water filter system. Filters for the showerhead are also very important.

Clean air and adequate sunshine are also important for adequate immune function and disease prevention. Air filters may be necessities for city dwellers.

Adequate Exercise

American extremes in exercise are like a college football game: twenty-two people beating their brains out on the field with eighty-thousand people sitting around watching. Some overdo it and many do nothing at all. Walking, swimming, cross-country machines, or mini trampolines may offer the most overall benefits. Any exercise you like to do is better than none. Dancing, racquetball, and other participatory sports are increasingly popular for the fun they add to movement. Remember: Even five to ten minutes of walking or any exercise is a fine beginning. Bowling, touch football, walking the dog more frequently—anything that gets you moving is worthwhile. Don't let an all-or-nothing approach stop you before you start.

Get Enough Rest
Sleep adequately. If you need an alarm to wake you, you are not getting enough rest. Go to bed as early as possible and sleep until you wake refreshed. Exercise and good nutrition help the body sleep more deeply.

Eat According to Individual Needs
We all have unique biochemistries. When the media tells you to eat a low-fat diet, take calcium, or eat a lot of carbohydrates, its prescriptions may run counter to your body's nutritional needs. Everything in your diet must be customized. That usually requires the guidance of a nutritionist or nutritionally oriented doctor, but is well worth the visit or two it takes to get you on the right track.

Nutrition Is Celebratory
Optimal health is not the result of deprivation. It celebrates the benefits of many foods and nutrients, allowing us more of life and health. It is the marriage of science and pleasure. Balance the information to your own best advantage. Discard that which is too difficult and use that which suits you. Don't try to be perfect or avoid all of your favorite foods, even if some of them are "bad." Improve your diet and lifestyle at whatever pace is best for you. Improving your health this way will only add to your enjoyment of life.

CHAPTER 2

What Is a Healthy Diet?

WE WALK THROUGH THE SUPERMARKET as if it were a mine-field. Food has become the enemy. We have our list of subversive food elements, and do our best to avoid them. We do everything to avoid fat, cholesterol, and the dangerous food of the day.

Eating less fat and food additives is not a bad idea. A healthy diet, however, is not arrived at by process of elimination. It is assembled from the foods with the most beneficial substances. More often than not, it is what we fail to eat that causes health problems, not merely what we do eat.

Before we can get a grasp of the elements of a healthy diet, the food industry takes advantage of our confusion. Foods are marketed not on the basis of what they have, but of what they lack. Sugar and white flour are mixed together with toxic additives to create cakes that are "fat-free." Margarine—a destructive food if ever there was one—is sold to you under the guise of being "cholesterol-free." And fried corn chips are celebrated for having "one-third less salt."

THE NEW APPROACH: EATING FOOD FOR WHAT IT HAS

- While eating less fat is good, getting the full range of nutrients needed to handle fat is better.
- Eating less sugar is beneficial, but get the fiber, B vitamins, and minerals like zinc and chromium needed to metabolize the small amounts of sugar you do eat.
- Avoid cholesterol only if it is oxidized. Oxidized cholesterol is found in processed foods or results in the body

when there is a lack of antioxidant nutrients. Oxidized cholesterol is found in powdered milk, scrambled or powdered eggs, mass-produced cakes and cake mixes, aged cheese, and aged meats such as sausages and aged steaks. Cholesterol in boiled eggs, fresh meat, and seafood is harmless when accompanied by vitamins C, E, beta-carotene, and a healthy diet.

The end of confusion in nutrition comes only when we understand the basic principles of healthy eating. Adopting these principles, we will find that everything—even a lot of the so-called conflicting information—falls into place.

THE PRINCIPLES OF HEALTHY EATING

- Eat whole, unrefined foods high in nutrient density and as close to their natural state as possible.
- Eat as wide a variety of foods as possible.
- Eat a diet that promoted longevity in your ancestors.
- Eat according to the needs of your own unique biochemistry and lifestyle.

You may be more surprised by what is not on this list than what is on it. Shouldn't we lower our fat intake? Eating foods close to their natural state will do that to the degree that it is necessary. What about decreasing sugar intake? Whole, unrefined foods are low in sugar. How much protein? Your ancestors' diet and the requirements of your own biochemistry dictate more about your protein needs than the current nutrition fad of the day.

Healthy eating principles don't lead to a restrictive, boring diet. Bland food is not necessarily health-promoting. Herbs, spices, condiments, and interesting ways of preparing foods are often beneficial. Many herbs we use to flavor foods are actually important sources of trace minerals and immune-boosting pigments known as bioflavonoids.

Eat Foods as Close to Their Natural State as Possible
Foods closest to their natural state are those richest in nutrients. The most delicate vitamins and essential fatty acids are those that we lack. They are also the ones missing from refined foods. Food manufacturers are interested in shelf life, not your life. They destroy or remove the delicate nutrients that have a tendency to spoil so their products can last for months or even

years on a supermarket shelf. To get plenty of these life-extending nutrients, stick to organic produce, whole grains, nuts, seeds, lean meat, or wild game. Wild game is very low in fat and much richer in essential fatty acids than the meat from farm-raised cattle.

The Problems with "Enriched" White Bread and White Flour Products

Whole-grain bread used to be called "the staff of life." In the 1890s, widespread refining of grain products began in America, and bread would never be the same. Nutrient-rich whole grains are rarely consumed by most Americans, who are hooked on the white "enriched" flours that have been stripped of their essential fatty acids, and most of their vitamins and minerals. They are also bleached and treated with other chemicals. These flours are called "enriched" because after thirty or more nutrients are removed during milling, four are added back. If someone took $30,000 from you and then gave you $4,000, would you feel enriched?

"Enriched" flours are:

- Much lower in zinc, manganese, chromium, B_6, and other valuable nutrients found in whole grains.
- Low in fiber. Fiber prevents a wide range of diseases and promotes healthy digestive function.
- Bromated, a process that leaves chemical residues that suppress thyroid function.
- Devoid of essential fatty acids. Whole grains supply small amounts of valuable omega-3 fats.
- Fortified with synthetic iron, the sole mineral added back to white flour. The body has a more difficult time limiting the absorption of synthetic iron. More can be absorbed than is needed, forming free radicals in the body. When Sweden began fortifying its flours with iron, liver cancer rates tripled.[4, 5]

Eat Nutrient-Dense Foods

The nutrient density of a food is the amount of vitamins, minerals, essential fatty acids, and protein it has relative to its caloric content. The more nutrient-dense, the more health-promoting a food is. These foods are those closest to their natural state as well.

- Fruits and vegetables, particularly those that are organically grown, are high in vitamins, minerals, and polyphenols, and are low in calories. Organic produce is the most nutrient-dense food known.
- Nuts and seeds are foods richest in minerals and contain valuable essential fatty acids. They are very nutrient-dense.
- Whole grains are nutrient-dense. Avoid white "enriched" flour, which is not.
- Nutrient-dense virgin flaxseed oil is rich in omega-3s, vitamin E, lecithin, phytosterols, and other beneficial nutrients. Supermarket vegetable oils are stripped of their beneficial substances, contain toxic trans fats, and lack nutrient density.
- Baked sliced sweet potato is extraordinarily nutrient-dense. Diet potato chips are junk. No matter how low in calories they are, they are still nutrient-poor.
- Fat-free processed cakes and cookies are not nutrient-dense.

The best way to assess food's value is to ask whether it has nutrient density. It is much more important than fat, cholesterol, or calorie content. Nutrient density balances the positive and negative aspects of food to give you the true picture of a food's impact on your body. It also makes you aware of beneficial nutrients you might have missed in higher-calorie, extremely health-promoting foods like raw nuts and virgin oils.

Don't be afraid of the caloric nature of foods like raw nuts, particularly raw almonds and fresh walnuts, or of beneficial oils such as virgin flaxseed oil. Raw nuts are an excellent source of magnesium, zinc, potassium, vitamin E, fiber, and unprocessed essential fatty acids, all of which Americans lack. For nuts to be beneficial, they must be fresh, kept refrigerated, and shelled immediately before eating. Organic nuts are highly recommended, as fat-rich foods like nuts concentrate the pesticides that are sprayed on them.

Studies of groups such as the Seventh Day Adventists show that eating nuts can significantly reduce the incidence of heart disease. Nuts should be eaten raw. Almonds may be soaked for a few hours to make them easier to digest. They should not be roasted in oil or even dry-roasted. High heat turns their beneficial oils into harmful substances, and destroys essential fatty acids and vitamins as well.

Eat a Wide Variety of Food

There are many advantages to eating as wide a variety of food as possible:

- Varying the foods you eat will give you a balanced intake of the wide selection of nutrients needed for optimal health. Eating the same four or five foods over and over again creates nutrient imbalances and deficiencies. No food has the perfect balance of nutrients that is found in a wide and varied diet. If you eat meat, seafood, and dairy products as your only sources for protein and avoid nuts and seeds, you may get plenty of zinc, but not enough copper. A lack of copper increases the risk of heart disease. Zinc and copper should be kept in optimal balance through a varied diet. Work with a nutritionist to determine your individual needs.

- Eating the same foods over and over again increases the chances that food allergies or intolerances may develop. Wheat and bread products, milk and dairy products, and oranges and citrus fruits are foods many of us eat every day. These are foods that many people have developed sensitivities to. This has much to do with the fact that they are eaten too often in our culture. Eating different foods decreases the chances that the immune system or intestinal tract may get "sick" of you eating the same food every day. One should ideally not eat the same food until four days have passed. In other words, try to have cheeses on Monday, then Friday. Have almonds Monday, walnuts Tuesday, hazelnuts Wednesday, etc. Have wheat Monday, oats Tuesday, brown rice Wednesday, etc.

- Eating a food every day that is not organically grown—cantaloupe, for example—exposes you to larger doses of pesticides than may be safe. According to the EPA, pesticides on cantaloupe are only safe when an adult eats no more than six cantaloupes per year. While organic cantaloupe is a wonderful source of beta-carotene, potassium, and vitamin C, chemically grown produce has residues that make it less desirable. Heavily sprayed produce like fruits and berries, especially strawberries, should be rotated in the diet as much as possible. Produce from foreign countries where pesticides like DDT may be used should be avoided.

Find Your Traditional Diet

Studies have shown that we are best suited to the type of diet our ancestors ate for thousands of years. People from China or India may do well on a diet high in starches because that is what they have been eating for centuries. Europeans are not always suited to such a regime. They often develop problems with their immune systems, energy levels, and skin when put on a high-carbohydrate, low-protein diet. They require more protein, less starch, and enough essential fatty acids, or they will not be healthy.

If you can find out what was unique about your ancestors' diet, you will discover what is unique about you. Native Americans of Vancouver, British Columbia, ate salmon as a staple in their diet for hundreds of years. Then a dam was built that destroyed the salmon population. After their dietary source for omega-3 fatty acids EPA and DHA was eliminated, their rate of schizophrenia more than doubled. Their rates of diabetes, alcoholism, migraines, arthritis, and depression increased as well. EPA and DHA are essential nutrients for them. Which nutrients are uniquely required by you and people of your ancestry?

The importance of ancestral influence is rarely appreciated by nutrition researchers today. A diet that helps one group of people is assumed to be beneficial for everyone. Peruvian Indians or rural Chinese may thrive on a low-fat, high-carbohydrate diet, but Eskimos would need to be hospitalized if they were put on it. The Chinese have livers that can metabolize protein more efficiently than those of Europeans or Africans. This explains why they may do better with less protein than other groups. You need to know where you came from in order to know what to eat.

Will a well-meaning nutritionist return from Mars one day proclaiming that uranium protects Martians from heart disease—and then suggest we eat it?

Customizing Your Diet

Other factors that will affect your individual needs:

- Environmental Stress: Exposures to toxins in the environment and diet
- Personal Stress: emotional and physical
- Activity Level

Both environmental and personal stress will increase your needs for protein as well as for essential fatty acids. These are two nutrients that help the body detoxify and nourish the nervous system when extra demands are placed upon it. Protective nutrients that also should be increased in times of stress include vitamin C, B complex, vitamin E, magnesium, zinc, and essential fatty acids from foods such as flaxseed oil.

Those who exercise vigorously will also need to ensure that they are getting a full array of antioxidants such as vitamin C and E to protect their tissues. Exercise has also been found to increase the need for chromium. They will also need more calories to balance the amount that they burn off. For some athletes with high muscle mass, as much as six thousand calories per day may be needed.

Macronutrients. The main elements in your eating program are protein, fat, and carbohydrates. Before we put them together, let's consider each one of these macronutrients separately.

Protein. Protein is found in lean meats, fowl, seafood, eggs, and dairy products. Lentils, beans, and grains like quinoa and amaranth have significant amounts of protein, although these foods are mostly starch. Nuts, nut butters, and seeds are also excellent sources for protein, but they are highest in beneficial fats.
Animal proteins are not all the same:

- Freshly prepared wild game — such as venison, wild buffalo, and game birds — is best. It is free of antibiotics, hormones, and pesticide residues and is as low as 7% fat. The fat it does contain is higher in essential fatty acids, including the valuable omega-3s.
- Farm-raised meat has up to 40% fat or more, and is much lower in essential fatty acids. It also contains antibiotic, hormone, and pesticide residues.
- Prepared or aged meats such as bologna, turkey roll, sausages, and aged steaks are the worst form of meat. These meat products often contain salt, nitrates, and other harmful preservatives. Worst of all, they are high in oxidized cholesterol, the harmful kind found only in processed animal products. How harmful? A recent study of 120,000 men and women showed those who consumed processed meats had a 72% higher risk for developing cancer while those who ate fresh meat had no increased risk.

When people tell you that meat is bad for you, ask them which meats they are referring to. Lean meats, especially wild game, are nothing but beneficial when consumed in an overall healthy diet rich in essential nutrients.

What Kind of Fat? The kind and quality of fat you eat is more important than the amount you eat. There are three kinds of fat:

- Saturated fats are those that are solid at room temperature: the fat in most meats and animal and dairy products, as well as coconut and palm oils.
- Unsaturated fats are those that are liquid at room temperature: virgin flax, olive, canola, sunflower, corn, and all unhydrogenated and unrefined vegetable oils, and fish oils.
- Toxic fats: margarines, vegetable shortenings, partially hydrogenated oils, fried oils used in very high-heat recipes, and refined junk oils sold in supermarkets.

Saturated fats have been accused but never conclusively shown to cause disease. The Finns eat a diet high in saturated fat and have a high rate of heart disease, while the Japanese have the lowest intake of saturated fat and have a low rate of heart disease. Yet the Eskimos have the highest level of saturated fat intake and have the lowest rate of heart disease of any people group. There are also many African tribes in which saturated fat consumption is high and heart disease rates are low. Just because some groups who eat saturated fats have high rates of heart disease does not prove saturated fat is a problem. In 1910 coronary artery disease was very rare when animal fat made up a much larger percentage of the fat in our diet.

Unsaturated liquid oils are beneficial, but only when consumed in small amounts and not refined and stripped of their nutrients. Excessive consumption of refined vegetable oils, particularly omega-6 oils such as safflower, sunflower, and corn oils, has been implicated in increasing the rates of heart disease, cancer, and obesity. Unrefined oils, however, particularly omega-3 oils such as canola and flaxseed oil, are rich sources of essential fatty acids that promote health and prevent disease.

Some fats are conditionally essential. For the Native Americans of British Columbia, EPA and DHA are essential. They may also be essential for arthritics and people with inflammatory or autoimmune diseases. For people who have low thyroid, have missing nutrients in their diet, eat margarine or fried foods, or have low levels of certain enzymes, another unsaturated fat known as GLA is essential.

What Kind of Carbohydrates? There are two types of carbohydrates, simple and complex. Simple carbohydrates are sugars found in fruits and fruit juices, vegetables, the lactose in milk, and the sucrose from beet and cane sugar. Complex carbohydrates are found in grains, beans, and legumes. Complex carbohydrates are by far the more beneficial, for they are digested more slowly. Sugars, juices, and sweet fruits should be limited as much as possible. They stress the glandular, immune, and hormonal systems of the body.

Carbohydrate-rich foods come from nature in health-promoting forms, but can be refined into less desirable foods:

- Whole apples—a good source of fiber, vitamins and minerals, and a valuable bioflavonoid called quercitin.
- Apple juice—devoid of fiber, quercitin, and much lower in vitamins and minerals. Because of the lack of fiber and potassium, the sugar in apple juice enters our system much more quickly and is more stressful to our body than eating whole apples.
- Concentrated apple juice used as a sweetener in baked products—a highly concentrated source of calories, devoid of vitamins and minerals. No different from any other form of sugar.

Basic Types of Diets

The Caveman Diet. This diet consists predominately of protein, small amounts of carbohydrates, and moderate amounts of fat. This diet has been of benefit to those with carbohydrate addiction, adrenal exhaustion, and those who have difficulty losing weight. It is also helpful for problems such as yeast overgrowth, low thyroid, low blood sugar, and high insulin levels. It is a diet that was popularized by Robert Atkins, M.D., for well over twenty years in more than five books. It is the predominant diet that has been used at his busy New York clinic on over ten thousand patients with many excellent results.

Many people do not tolerate carbohydrates well. They are addicted to them. Unless carbohydrates are severely limited, they overeat or develop yeast overgrowth in their intestinal tracts, and excess weight and low energy levels may result.

This diet is called the "Caveman Diet" because for thousands of years before the development of agriculture, mankind had only two food groups: wild game and vegetation. This has led many researchers to feel that a higher intake of protein and lower intake of starches may be more optimal than the high-carbohydrate diet currently promulgated by the media.

The Caveman Diet, however, may not be optimal for everyone. Those with kidney disease and osteoporosis should restrict protein. Those of Asian descent of also often do better on a diet higher in starches and lower in protein.

The High-Carbohydrate/Low-Fat Diet. This diet has been popularized of late by Dr. John McDougall and Dr. Dean Ornish. This diet emphasizes grains, beans, and legumes, and keeps fat consumption to an absolute minimum. Protein is also restricted to as little as 20% of the diet. It was the late Nathan Pritikin who first recognized that a diet high in starches has the ability to lower cholesterol and regress arterial plaque in some people. However, other people's cholesterol levels will rise on a high-carbohydrate diet. While some may thrive on this diet, many do not fare well on it in the long term. A diet high in carbohydrates increases blood levels of the hormone insulin. High insulin levels are one of the strongest risk factors for heart disease.[6, 7]

Those of Chinese or Indian descent may find this high-carbohydrate diet appropriate and in keeping with their ancestral eating patterns. Those who wish to be vegetarians will also opt for this approach. Yet for many people, a diet that is 70% carbohydrates will lead to food cravings and weight gain. This is particularly true for women over forty who require more protein and fat in their diet to balance blood sugar and hormones. People who stay on this regime for long periods of time may develop skin and immune problems, fatigue, yeast overgrowth, PMS, and food cravings. For a complete discussion of problems of high carbohydrate diets, read Ann Louise Gittleman's classic *Beyond Pritikin*.

A More Balanced Approach

Recent evidence suggests that the best diet for overall health as well as weight loss is one that is approximately 30% protein,

30% fat, and 40% carbohydrates, while also abundant in vitamins, minerals, and essential fatty acids. This balance of macronutrients appears to have the best effect on keeping blood sugar, insulin, and prostaglandins balanced. Prostaglandins are the most powerful hormonal system in the human body. Keeping them in balance is essential for optimal health.[8]

This diet will not suit everyone. Some thrive on a diet of grains and beans and feel sensational when they eat as little fat as possible. Others will feel tired, get colds often, and have dry skin if they do not include their daily dose of healthy fats. And still others need to restrict their carbohydrates in order to feel wonderful. Yet for most people the balanced approach works best.

You Are Unique

An unexamined diet is not worth eating. Do your best to understand what ratio of carbohydrates to fat to protein will work best for you. No matter what the latest diet is or what someone tells you from his/her experience, your metabolism has unique needs. There are no absolute rules in nutrition, no laws, just principles. The diet that works best for you may be something along the lines of the balanced regime above. It may also be something completely different. Your metabolism is as unique as your personality. Whether you work with a nutritionist or experiment on your own, create a program that suits you best.

CHAPTER 3

What Is a Carbohydrate?

CARBOHYDRATES ARE FOODS THAT ARE rich in sugars or complexes of sugars. How the sugars are arranged will determine whether we call a food a source of **simple** or **complex carbohydrates**. Fruits and sugars are simple carbohydrates because they contain easily digested sugars. When sugars are bound into rows, as they are in starches such as whole grains and legumes, they are called complex carbohydrates. Just as it takes you much longer to know a complicated person, it takes the body much longer to digest the sugar from a complex carbohydrate.

Simple Carbohydrates	Complex Carbohydrates
White sugar	Whole Grains: whole wheat, oats, brown rice
Succanat (dehydrated cane juice)	Corn, peas, whole-grain pasta
White flour, white rice, white corn grits	Lentils and beans (navy, pinto, etc.)
Honey, barley malt, maple syrup, milk sugar	Leafy green vegetables
Fruits and fruit juices	Tubers: potatoes, onions, turnips

Most of the benefits attributed to carbohydrate foods come from the slower-digesting, complex variety. Complex carbohydrates are, in general, better because they take longer to digest. The sugars in these foods enter the body more slowly. They do not cause the sharp increase in blood sugar that can be caused by simple carbohydrates, especially sugars such as white sugar, honey, and other concentrated sweeteners. Even fruit, as bountiful as it is in vitamins and minerals and fiber, should not be viewed as a food that can be eaten with abandon. More than three servings of fruit per day has been found to raise triglyceride levels in sedentary people. A higher intake of fruit is only appropriate for the very active.

Carbohydrate foods in their natural state have many benefits: They are high in fiber, low in fat, and a good source of vitamins. They can also be a good source of minerals, depending on the mineral content of the soil they were grown in. Carbohydrates, like any food or nutrient, however, are only beneficial in the right amount. If you want to derive all the benefits of carbohydrates, you need to eat them in the amount that is right for you.

Americans need to eat more of the complex variety. More than three quarters of the carbohydrates we consume come from refined sugars and flours.

When sugars or starches become a larger percentage of our diet than best suits our individual biochemistry, carbohydrate toxicity occurs. Carbohydrate toxicity is increasingly widespread due to the following misconceptions circulated by the media:

- The more carbohydrates you eat, the better.
- All carbohydrates are created equal.
- All fat is bad and should be avoided as much as possible.
- We eat too much protein and need to eat less.

None of the preceding is true. The problem with this erroneous nutritional belief system is that it leads one to overload the body with carbohydrates, and the following problems result:

- Excess carbohydrate intake displaces protein, which is needed for energy, tissue repair, blood sugar balance, and immune function.
- Excessive carbohydrate intake will lead to excessive levels of insulin, which can cause weight gain, bloating, fatigue, food cravings, and cardiovascular disease.
- Faddish high-carbohydrate, ultra-low-fat diets do not provide enough essential fatty acids.

- Too many carbohydrates, especially concentrated sweeteners, can stress the adrenal glands into a state of exhaustion.
- Diets too high in carbohydrates upset prostaglandins, a family of hormonelike compounds that must be in balance for health to exist.[9]
- A diet too high in carbohydrates and too low in protein can cause liver damage.

The right amount of carbohydrates for most people is about 40% of their diet, with emphasis on the complex variety. More than 50% of the diet as carbohydrates or too many refined carbohydrates causes problems. Complex carbohydrates in the right amount are beneficial. Those who refine and overeat them bring out their bad side. Too much of anything is bad for the body, and low-fat starchy foods are no exception.

While the preceding percentages are a helpful guide, the optimal intake of carbohydrates will differ for each person. Some may thrive on a diet that consists mostly of carbohydrates. Most, however, will not. Many women over age thirty will feel bloated and tired on a diet that is 60% carbohydrates or more. We are all different, and need to examine our own unique metabolism to determine our optimal range for carbohydrate intake.

METABOLIZING CARBOHYDRATES

All carbohydrate foods are eventually broken down into sugar and put into your bloodstream. Your body has a system of glands that helps you balance your blood sugar. If this system is healthy, then carbohydrates can be eaten freely as part of a balanced diet. If this system is damaged, as it often is by coffee, sugar, alcohol, cigarettes, a lack of sleep, and the effects of stress and a nutrient-depleted diet, then more than 40% of the diet as carbohydrates may cause problems. Other factors that weaken the body's carbohydrate-handling mechanisms include:

- High insulin levels
- Low blood sugar
- Obesity
- Female hormone imbalance/PMS
- Inactivity
- Heredity
- Low thyroid function

- Diabetes
- Candida overgrowth
- Food allergies

High Insulin Levels

Insulin is a hormone that is secreted from the pancreas, especially when we eat. When carbohydrate foods are eaten, we secrete the most insulin. High insulin levels may be one of the factors that cause heart disease and obesity, and chronically high insulin leads to adult-onset diabetes. A balanced diet that is moderate in carbohydrates—predominately the complex variety—will keep insulin in a healthy range, especially when accompanied by enough zinc and chromium. Too many carbohydrates, especially refined carbohydrates, along with a shortage of these minerals will elevate insulin.

Obesity

Persons who are significantly overweight often have higher blood levels of insulin. Because insulin is involved in stimulating the storage of carbohydrates as fat, high insulin levels can make weight loss difficult. Many obese people with high insulin levels require a diet that is no more than 40% carbohydrates. They also benefit from supplements of insulin-metabolizing trace minerals chromium and zinc.

Tired Adrenal Glands

Your adrenals are walnut-sized glands that sit atop your kidneys and perform many tasks in order to keep you alert and healthy. One of their most important jobs is to keep blood sugar balanced. If you have been eating a lot of sugar, white flour, fruit juices, coffee, and alcohol over an extended period of time, your adrenal glands' ability to keep blood sugar stable will be weakened. If you are tired all the time and do not have the energy you used to, see a nutritionally oriented health professional who can help you assess the strength of your adrenals. Fatigue can be due to many things, but tired adrenals are almost always involved.

If you do have tired adrenals, you have more reason to stick to a diet that is moderate in carbohydrates. Putting a person with exhausted blood-sugar-balancing glands on a high-carbohydrate diet is like taking a car with broken shocks over a bumpy road. You are going to bounce all over the place. Those with exhausted glands will do best to stick to a diet balanced in protein, carbohydrates, and essential fatty acids.

Hypoglycemia

Low blood sugar is another condition that will usually not benefit from a diet high in carbohydrates. Persons with hypoglycemia can benefit from certain starchy foods like beans and legumes, which release their sugars very slowly and are a great help at balancing blood sugar. But all simple sugars and even more than two servings of fruit can cause hypoglycemics to tire. Again, moderation with carbohydrates is key.

ARE VEGETARIAN DIETS FOR EVERYONE?

Vegetarian diets are typically high in carbohydrates. Although vegetarian diets are high in protective vitamins such as beta-carotene, vitamin C, and folic acid, as well as fiber, such regimes do not offer enough B_{12} if all animal foods are avoided. Scientists have found that vegetarian societies have difficulty adapting to stress. This may be due to low levels of the amino acids methionine, threonine, and tryptophan in the vegetarian diet. While a vegetarian or macrobiotic regime may suit some people, eliminating all sources of concentrated animal protein may not suit hypoglycemics, people with adrenal burnout, persons with hypothyroid, and those with yeast overgrowth. The lacto-ovo vegetarian diet, that is, a vegetarian diet that includes eggs and dairy products, appears to be the most beneficial form of vegetarianism.

Whether meat and poultry consumption is healthful or not will depend on our genetics, lifestyle/stress level, and the other foods and nutrients that are present in the diet. While the quality of the meat you consume is important, other factors in your diet will play a large part in determining the effect of meat on your body.

- Meat contains a significant amount of iron. This is often beneficial for children and menstruating and pregnant women, but potentially harmful for men and postmenopausal women.
- Most meat contains significant amounts of fat, which, combined with the iron in meat, damages the intestinal wall. The degree to which this occurs depends on the rest

of your diet. If you consume significant amounts of anti-oxidants, produce or supplements, have a high fiber intake, and maintain beneficial bacteria in your colon through the use of bifidobacterium and FOS food supplements (see Chapter 20), you will prevent this damage from occurring. Yet if vitamins, vegetables, and high-fiber foods are not a part of your diet and you have never done anything to encourage healthy bacteria in your GI tract, then the negative effects of meat can go a long way toward eroding your health.

- The quality of the meat you consume is also important. Aged meat is a definite no-no, for it is high in toxins such as malonaldehyde. Aged meat is carcinogenic while fresh meat is not. Low-fat meats are also preferable, such as wild game, lean cuts like flank steak, white-meat turkey, and skinless free-range chicken.

Lean cuts of meat can be an important source of zinc, protein, and other nutrients. As part of a balanced diet, meat can be health-promoting, particularly wild game. In general, try to get meat from animals that were fed organic feed and raised without hormones or antibiotics.

The worst thing about meat is what it does to the planet. It takes much more resources to create a pound of meat than a pound of grain. Destruction of the rain forest is occurring at a staggering rate around the world. Much of this land is being cleared to allow cattle more grazing room. Keep meat consumption moderate, and balance it with complex carbohydrates found in beans, legumes, and whole grains, moderate amounts of fruit, and the good fats found in virgin flaxseed and olive oils, raw nuts, and seeds.

Summing Up

- Each of us has different carbohydrate needs.
- Complex carbohydrates, found in vegetables, whole grains, beans, and legumes, are best.
- Limit fruit and fruit juices to a maximum of three servings per day unless you do a significant amount of exercise.
- Our needs for carbohydrates will change throughout our lives, decreasing as we get older.

- Sedentary people need less carbohydrates than those who exercise regularly.
- Make sure that you are eating at least two meals per day that contain significant amounts of protein.
- A higher intake of carbohydrates will increase your need for B vitamins, zinc, and chromium.
- Bloating, fatigue, or sugar or starch cravings are a sign that you may be consuming excessive quantities of carbohydrates.
- Consult a nutritionist for the best plan to suit your individual needs.
- For most people, 40% of calories as carbohydrates is best.

CHAPTER 4

Are All Fats Bad for You?

Beware of false knowledge; it is more dangerous than ignorance.
—G. B. Shaw

IF YOU BELIEVE THE NUTRITION media, nearly every health problem we have today is caused by too much fat in our diet. If we only ate less, all our health problems would go away. Not true. There are really three problems with fat, and they have very little to do with the quantity of fat we eat:

- We consume too many nonessential fats and not enough essential fats.
- We eat fats and oils that are too refined and dangerously altered.
- We do not consume the wide range of nutrients the body needs to handle fat correctly.

Americans eat an average of sixty-three pounds of fat a year. Lowering fat consumption is not a bad idea, but alone would have little impact on the epidemic of diseases such as heart disease and cancer. Fat consumption went down 2% from 1978 to 1990 while the rates of obesity and degenerative diseases increased. We do not need to eat less fat. We need to eat better fats and a diet abundant in essential nutrients.

What we do not understand, we fear. Because Americans do not understand how fat functions as part of a healthy diet, they are afraid of it. Our media has further fueled this paranoia. The results?

- Fat-free, sugar-laden junk foods are hawked as beneficial snacks.
- A lack of health-generating essential fatty acids of the omega-3 class in our diet, which can lead to a weakened, imbalanced immune system and an increased risk of degenerative diseases.

44

- Foods high in protein and fat are avoided, and more refined carbohydrates are eaten instead, leading to an unhealthy dietary imbalance. This increases the incidence of hypoglycemia, PMS, and obesity.

Too Much of Anything Is Bad

Too much fat is a problem, but so is too much brown rice, exercise, or water. Anything in excess is unhealthy. We should all eat less fat, perhaps 30% of our diet. But quality is much more important than quantity. Refined and altered fats are bad. Unprocessed fats and oils are not when consumed in moderation as part of a healthy diet.[10, 11]

What to Ask About the Fat You Eat

- What kind of fat is it (essential/nonessential)?
- Has it, like most supermarket oils, been stripped of all its nutrients? Or is it rich in vitamins, phytosterols, lecithin, and essential fatty acids, as are virgin flaxseed and canola oils from responsible manufacturers?
- Is it sold in glass, which allows light to damage oil, or is it sold in opaque containers that preserve the oil's freshness?
- Is it organic? Does it have pesticide or other chemical residues?
- Am I consuming fat in a balance with other macronutrients, such as protein and fiber?
- Do I have an optimal intake of vitamins and minerals in order to have a healthy fat metabolism?

Fat Is Essential

If you removed all the fat from your body, you would die instantly. Your cell membranes and nervous system would collapse. Don't think of fat as harmful unless you are referring to processed fats such as margarine, fried foods, and commercially produced vegetable oils that have had their vitamin E removed. These are bad fats. Fat in its natural state, unadulterated by man, and consumed in moderate amounts as part of a balanced diet rich in all essential nutrients, has yet to be proven "bad."

Fat's Many Valuable Roles
- Essential fatty acids boost the immune system and ward off disease.
- Fat helps slow the release of sugar into your bloodstream, important for hypoglycemics and diabetics.
- Fat does not feed fungal overgrowths as carbohydrates do.
- Fat is needed for the absorption of vitamins A, E, D, K, and beta-carotene.
- Fat is needed to form all cell membranes.

ESSENTIAL AND NONESSENTIAL FATTY ACIDS

Of all the fats we consume, two fatty acids are essential. They are linoleic acid (an omega-6 fatty acid) and alpha-linolenic acid (an omega-3 fatty acid). Omega-6 linoleic can be found in all vegetable oils and most grains and beans. Omega-3 alpha-linolenic is found in fewer foods: flaxseed and flax oil, fresh walnuts and walnut oil, chia seeds, pumpkin seeds, and soy and canola oils. If we do not receive both of these fatty acids on a regular basis, our health will deteriorate.

THE REFINING OF FATS

Commercially manufactured liquid vegetable oils in the United States are refined to an extraordinary degree. They are heated, deodorized, and have many valuable nutrients removed. The vitamin E that is present in unrefined vegetable oils is taken out and sold to the vitamin industry. The lecithin that helps our body emulsify and use fats more effectively is removed. The result is a naked oil that is nearly devoid of nutritional value. It is then stored in clear glass that light can penetrate, damaging the oil. It is hard to imagine a commercial process for oil manufacturing that could be worse.

But there is one. It's called hydrogenation, and it turns liquid oils into solid, strange fats that do not fit into our metabolism. Hydrogenation is a process that places oils under tremendous pressure and high heat in the presence of hydrogen and metal catalysts. The hydrogenated oils that result are used to make margarine and shortenings, and are present in a wide variety of baked and snack foods. Cereals, candy, chips, cake mixes, and bread often contain these toxic fats. Hydrogenated oils do much of the damage we attribute to fat ingestion. In many of the studies in which saturated fats were said to cause disease, hydrogenated vegetable oil was actually the fat that was used. Many cultures have used saturated fats for thousands of years without ill effects. No culture has ever used hydrogenated vegetable oils without increasing their rates of disease.[12]

OILS MUST BE ORGANIC

Fats that come from heavily sprayed plants—such as the cotton plant—act as powerful carriers of all the pesticides that were sprayed on the crop. Pesticides are usually fat-soluble and have an affinity for the oils in the seeds of plants that are sprayed. Pesticides cause a wide variety of diseases. When you buy vegetable oils, do everything possible to ensure that the oil is from a plant that has not been sprayed with pesticides or fungicides. Make sure that the oil is certified organic. Otherwise you may be adding a significant source of pesticides to your diet.

BALANCE IS IMPORTANT

It is important to keep a good balance between essential and nonessential fats. Even if we are consuming one tablespoon of flaxseed oil per day, we can develop a *relative* deficiency of essential fats if we are consuming too many nonessential fats such as those found in other foods, be it the fats in meat, dairy products, or even almonds. These latter fats are not bad, but we must balance them with foods rich in essential fats such as canola and flaxseed oil, cold-water fish, and raw walnuts and pumpkin seeds.

Many Americans are consuming too many fats of the omega-6 class and not enough of the omega-3 family. Eating meat and safflower, sunflower, and corn oils fills the body with omega-6s. If no flaxseed oil, walnuts, salmon, sardines, or mackerel find their way into your diet, you will have no omega-3 fats to counter the pro-inflammatory effect of the omega-6s. Over a long period of time, this will increase your risk of inflammation and degenerative diseases. Balance among essential fatty acids is critical for long-term health.

Fat Has Three Roles in the Body

- **Structural:** It is incorporated into cell membranes and other body structures. It is used in fatty tissue that insulates and cushions the body.
- **Metabolic:** It can be changed into powerful hormones known as prostaglandins that profoundly affect metabolism.
- **Fuel:** It can be burned for energy.

Our cells membranes are like trading posts where sugar, hormones, protein, and other nutrients are exchanged. Healthy membrane function is essential for overall health. If our diet contains essential fatty acids found in virgin flaxseed, walnut, and canola oils, or those found in cold-water fish, our cells will remain flexible and healthy. When the wrong fats are consumed, such as margarines, fried foods, baked goods, or refined supermarket oils, or we have an inadequate intake of beneficial fats, cell membranes suffer. They become stiff or have holes in them, decreasing our health significantly and increasing our risk of degenerative disease.

Prostaglandins

An archer reaches into his quiver for an arrow that will go the distance. Your cells reach into the cell membrane for a fatty acid that will perform well when shot through the cell as a prostaglandin. Prostaglandins are hormones, and certain fatty acids are turned into them every moment you are alive. If the fat you eat is health-promoting, like flax oil, good prostaglandins will be made with beneficial effects upon your metabolism. If you consume mostly altered and refined fats and oils, the prostaglandins you make will have more inflammatory, immune-suppressing effects and your health will be compromised. Whether you are healthy or sick, it is largely because of the quality of your prostaglandins.

Flaxseed Oil. This is an oil that should be used in salad dressings and on cooked vegetables and baked potatoes. It should never be heated, although it can be placed on hot foods. Flax oil has the most omega-3 fats of any vegetable oil. It has been found to have a wide range of health-enhancing effects. It can lower cholesterol and triglycerides, has anti-inflammatory effects, and enhances immune function.

Canola Oil. Canola oil is another excellent food that contains essential fatty acids. It may be used for salads, baking, and low-heat recipes. In its unrefined, beneficial form, canola oil has a golden color and a pleasant taste.

Extra-Virgin Olive Oil. This is an excellent oil for many applications, from salads to sautéing. The green extra-virgin may have a strong taste, but is far more health-enhancing than the pure olive oil, which has had many beneficial substances removed.

Peanut Oil. Peanut oil can withstand higher temperatures better than most oils. It is the oil of choice for use in stir-fry cooking. Stir-frying with garlic, onions, red pepper, turmeric, and other spices helps to give the oil more stability under high heat.

The kind of fat you should buy, whether you are buying flax or canola oils, is oil that has been processed as minimally as possible. Only buy flaxseed and canola oils that are sold in opaque, black plastic containers. Light damages oil, and we need to consume oils that are damaged as little as possible if they are going to augment our health.

Fat only causes disease when:
- **Fats are refined or overly heated.** Fried fats, hydrogenated oils, and refined supermarket vegetable oils all deteriorate health.
- **Essential fatty acids are missing.** A lack of the goods fats weakens the body. That is why omega-3 rich virgin flaxseed and canola oils should be everyday foods.
- **There is an imbalance in essential fatty acids.** Too much omega-6, found in corn, sunflower, and safflower oils, and not enough omega-3, can cause health problems.
- **The body lacks the vitamins and minerals to metabolize fats correctly.** A diet of white flour, white sugar, and other empty calories deprives our body of the nutrients we need to metabolize fat correctly.
- **Excessive amounts of calories are consumed.** Studies have shown that as long as we eat a normal amount of calories, moderate consumption of fats and oils in their natural state will not promote disease.

Fats and oils in their natural state promote health. If we had never refined or altered them or refined the rest of our diet, fats would never have caused a problem.

Summing Up

- Get enough of the essential fats in your diet. The best way is with one to three tablespoons of virgin organic flax or canola oil per day.
- Avoid all refined supermarket vegetable oils sold in glass bottles. Virgin oils have a golden color, and should only be bought when sold in opaque containers.
- Eliminate white flour, sugar, and all fat-free "junk" foods from your diet.
- Avoid fried foods, margarine, and vegetable shortenings and the snack and baked foods that contain them.
- Eat plenty of fruits and vegetables and take supplemental vitamin C, E, and beta-carotene found in a good antioxidant formula.
- Exercise regularly, but not until three hours after any meal that is high in fat. When your blood is filled with fat from a recent meal, it cannot carry as much oxygen as the body needs for aerobic exercise.

Fat metabolism is like the electrical wiring in your house. If you have live wires (bad fat metabolism from missing nutrients), using no electricity—eating no fat—is not the answer. Fixing the wires—getting the right vitamins, minerals, and essential fatty acids your body needs to handle fat correctly—is the right choice.

CHAPTER 5

The Trouble with Margarine

You can't spell margarine without "angina."
—David Letterman

I F YOU ARE LIKE MOST Americans, you eat a significant amount of partially hydrogenated oils. These altered fats are found in your diet every day through margarine, vegetable shortening, cakes, cookies, crackers, chips, and an assortment of other baked, fried, and processed foods. Every time your body tries to create health, make prostaglandins, or perform duties in and around cell membranes, the hydrogenated oils you eat get in the way.

Hydrogenated oils are liquid oils that are turned solid through the addition of hydrogen, pressure, and metal catalysts like nickel. This process creates fatty acids known as trans fats that have wide-ranging destructive power. These new, and strange fatty acids walk through your body like Frankenstein, terrorizing your metabolism.

Hydrogenated oil products like margarine are rejected by animals. In one experiment, a stick of margarine was left on a windowsill for one year, and no life form would touch it. Birds have been known to reject hydrogenated oils. These altered fats are a plastic food that only humans can be tricked into eating.

We have known about the problems caused by margarine and other partially hydrogenated oils for decades. Outspoken researchers like Mary Enig, Ph.D., have pointed out the dangers of margarine for many years, yet only now are industry and the public beginning to listen. Dr. Enig and others have urged that all hydrogenated oils in margarine, shortening, and baked goods be removed from the food supply due to the widespread, long-term damage they cause.

Margarine, vegetable shortenings, and all hydrogenated oils:
- Raise total cholesterol levels 20–30 mg%.
- Lower HDL cholesterol and raise LDL cholesterol.
- Decrease quality of a mother's breast milk by lowering its fat content.
- Promote inflammation.
- Create higher levels of circulating insulin and may cause diabetes.
- Increase the number of fat cells and promote obesity.
- Reduce the ability of the body to rid itself of toxins, carcinogens, and drugs.
- Dangerously alter the function of cell membranes throughout the body.
- Decrease immune function.

AREN'T SATURATED FATS THE PROBLEM?

The innocent are found guilty and the dangerous walk free. Saturated fats, the solid fats found in meat and dairy products, are blamed for causing heart disease. In 1910 when coronary artery disease was very rare, animal fats constituted 83% of total fat intake, and liquid vegetable oils 17%. Today, animal fats make up 58% of the fat intake of Americans, and vegetable fat, much of it in the form of hydrogenated margarines and shortenings, constitutes a whopping 42%. Today, heart disease is epidemic. Saturated fats are not to blame. They are an essential part of your metabolism. If you ate no saturated fatty acids, your body would make them. However, the human body has never experienced the large intake of hydrogenated oils found in margarine until the twentieth century.

IS BUTTER BETTER THAN MARGARINE?

During World War II, Northern Europe had its supply of hydrogenated margarines and shortenings cut off and then witnessed the steepest decline in heart disease it has seen this century. Countries like Norway, Denmark, and Holland consumed the dairy products they once exported and increased their butter intake to 20 grams per day—five times the amount consumed in America today—with beneficial results. If you are looking for something to replace margarine with, look no further than butter.

Butter has been eaten in moderate amounts for thousands of years without causing health problems. As part of a diet rich in vitamins, minerals, fiber, and essential fatty acids, butter has no deleterious effects. Virgin olive and flax oil would be an even better choice for use on baked potatoes and cooked vegetables.

If you are looking for an oil to cook with, first try to switch to nonstick pans. Heating any oil is undesirable. Small amounts of coconut oil can be used to coat pans when needed. Coconut oil is perfectly suited to this task, because it withstands heat well without being turned into damaging substances. Coconut oil has saturated fats, but in small amounts and as part of a healthy diet, saturated fats are harmless. Saturated fats are exactly the fat to use in situations in which an oil has to be used to coat a pan.

Margarine consumption was demonstrated in a recent study to significantly increase the risk for coronary heart disease. How many studies will have to appear before we realize the insanity of using toxic fats on an everyday basis?[13]

Don't buy margarine because it doesn't have cholesterol. Gasoline doesn't either, and you don't spread that on your toast. Avoid margarine because of what it does have: the single most toxic substance in our food supply, trans fatty acids.

SUMMING UP

- Check all food labels for "partially hydrogenated vegetable oil" and "vegetable shortening." Anything using the word *hydrogenated* should be avoided. Be especially watchful of all baked products, breads, crackers, cookies, cereals, candy, cakes and cake mixes, donuts, frostings, chips, and mayonnaise.
- Avoid all fried foods, including French fries, fish fillets, and deep-fried entrées.
- Liquid vegetable oils that are in the supermarket may also contain trans fats. Switch instead to more responsibly made oils from the health food store. Virgin flax, canola, and olive oils are best.
- When dining out, tell your waiter that you do not want your food prepared or served with margarine.[14, 15, 16, 17]

CHAPTER 6

Is Sugar Bad for You?

Beware of sweet dainties; they are a deceitful food.

—Proverbs 23:3

YOU ARE A MAJOR LEAGUE baseball player standing at the plate. The pitcher goes into his windup. The next thing you know, three baseballs fly past you. You are out before you could even try to adapt.

That is exactly what happens to your body when you feed it sugar. The body was never designed to deal with the explosive effects of sugar. When you eat it, you stun and stress your organs and greatly increase your risk of developing every degenerative disease. On average, every American eats 133 pounds per year. This is one of the major causes for the epidemic levels of heart disease, adult-onset diabetes, immune dysfunction, and premature aging.

The problems with sugar are well documented in major medical journals worldwide. Yet we continue to ignore the warnings.

Sugar has been shown to:
- Increase the risk for breast cancer[18, 19]
- Double the risk for biliary tract cancer[20]
- Deplete B vitamins and chromium
- Interfere with the absorption of calcium and magnesium[21]
- Cause heart disease[22]
- Increase cholesterol and insulin levels[23, 24]
- Raise blood pressure[25]
- Raise triglycerides[26]
- Weaken the immune system[27, 28]
- Cause a deficiency of copper[29]
- Cause varicose veins[30]
- Damage the kidneys[31]

- Cause or worsen arthritis[32]
- Cause migraine headaches[33]
- Increase the acidity of the stomach
- Cause gallstones[34]
- Contribute to obesity[35]

The idea that sugar is bad goes against instinct. Our desire for sweetness is a natural sense that helped us in the wild by driving us away from poisonous, bitter foods and toward beneficial sweet foods such as corn, peas, carrots, and the occasional fruit. When we are in the wild, we can distinguish which foods are healthful by tasting them for their sweetness. Naturally sweet foods promote health by providing vitamins, valuable phenolic compounds, minerals, and trace amounts of essential fatty acids. Their rich fiber content slows the release of their sugar into our bloodstream, and their mineral content helps the body use sugar more effectively. In this setting, balanced by other nutrients found in whole foods, sugar is a natural part of a healthy diet.

But we can't leave well enough alone. If sweetness attracts us to a food, why not extract the sweet taste of sugar and put it on everything? Pure sugar will increase our desire for anything that it is put on. That is one of the reasons the processed food industry thrives today. Sugar makes toxic, refined foods taste good. Sugar bribes the body. It says, "Look, this really tastes good!" and the body goes along for the ride, taking in junk foods that it otherwise wouldn't. The result is a deterioration of health. Fruits and vegetables that contain sugar, when eaten as part of a balanced diet, build up the body. Purified sugars from these foods, however, destroy it.

I have counseled many people who feel tired and fatigued when they eat sugar. They often ask, "Why can't I eat sugar anymore? I used to eat it all the time and felt fine. Now it makes me feel exhausted. What's wrong with me?" Their bodies could never handle sugar. It strains the organs of the body, forcing reserve energy to be spent. After years of struggling to deal with the stress of sugar and assaults from coffee, stress, and a nutrient-depleted diet, the glands of the body give out. Such weakened metabolisms need to be especially careful to avoid all sweets, stimulants, and stresses, and to receive adequate protein, vitamins, minerals, and essential fatty acids every day.

How About Just Eating Less Sugar?

Eating less sugar is better. Eating no refined sweeteners is optimal. Eating sugar makes you want more sugar. It isn't easy to regulate your intake of it if you allow it in your diet at all. If you must eat sugary foods, have them only on special occasions, or at most, once per week. Sugar should ideally only be in your diet where it occurs in nature—in berries, fruit, carrots, sweet potatoes, and other produce rich in phenols, vitamins, minerals, and fiber.

When Your Blood Sugar Is Imbalanced, You Are, Too

Blood sugar keeps your brain and body on an even keel. When it is low or takes steep dives, you will feel light-headed, weak, and depressed. You will crave sugar in order to regain your energy. Blood sugar levels are kept in balance by the pancreas, adrenal glands, and other tissues, all of which are destroyed by purified sugar. Sugar is not a pick-me-up. It is a drag-you-down.

As sugar burns out our blood sugar balancing mechanisms, it makes us want more. We can no longer keep our own sugar levels balanced, and want sugar as often as possible to relieve depression or low energy levels. We are caught in a vicious circle. The way out is to avoid it completely.

Paralyzing the Immune System

Sugar paralyzes the immune system. When we are healthy and avoid sugar, our protective white blood cells circle the body like energetic prizefighters knocking out viruses and bacteria that create illness. Yet these same protective pugilists can be knocked unconscious by sugar—even the sugar found in a large glass of fruit juice. The immune-paralyzing effect of a dose of sugar equivalent to that found in twelve ounces of sweetened soda can last for up to five hours. If you are someone who frequently gets colds or has problems with your immune system, avoid sugar in all its forms. It is the first and most important strategy to employ to keep your immune system strong. Even carrot juice, as rich as it is in beta-carotene and other beneficial nutrients, can depress immune function with its high sugar content.

Sugar also depresses immune function by encouraging the overgrowth of a yeast organism known as candida albicans.

Candida is a yeast naturally present in small amounts in everyone's intestinal tract. But when sugar is consumed, candida may overgrow, leading to bloating, gas, depression, low energy levels, and a host of other problems. Sugar in and of itself does not always lead to candida overgrowth. Consuming sugar regularly, however, significantly increases the chances that the yeast organism known as candida albicans will change into its fungal form, overgrow in the GI tract and elsewhere in the body, and cause health problems.

"NATURAL" SUGARS

Natural does not mean health-promoting. Crude oil is natural, yet ten million gallons of it killed an enormous amount of wildlife in Prince William Sound, Alaska. Celebrating "unrefined sweeteners" as natural is misleading. Honey, maple syrup, rice syrup, and barley malt are all no less of a source of refined carbohydrates than white sugar. Concentrated fruit juice has none of the goodness of fruit left in it. While slightly less draining on the adrenal system than white sugar, these sweeteners are just as bad at raising cholesterol and triglycerides, depressing immune function, and causing candida overgrowth. Use them only as a transition away from white sugar and toward a diet that has no refined sugars of any kind.

CAN'T WE HAVE IT NOW AND THEN?

In small amounts, sweeteners may pose little risk for people who are otherwise healthy. Yet eating sugar is like hitting yourself in the head with a baseball bat. The less you do it, the better. Sugar always stresses the body. Healthy persons may not initially feel this stressing effect, but will eventually. By the time you feel it, it may be too late. Sugar may have claimed you as another victim of its subtle and destructive effects.

BUT I HAVE FRIENDS WHO EAT SUGAR AND THEY LOOK HEALTHY . . .

Those who eat sugar with no outwardly visible effects do not prove sugar is innocuous any more than a survivor of Russian roulette proves that game's safety. Remember: If sugar is clogging your arteries, suppressing your immune system, and exhausting your adrenal glands and pancreas, you won't know until it is too late. If you are someone who has been burned out by sugar, do your best to follow the healthy eating guidelines outlined in this book. Get plenty of chromium, zinc, and adequate amounts of protein throughout the day. Use tonics like standardized ginseng extract to strengthen your sugar-balancing adrenal glands. Count to ten before you get angry, employ relaxation techniques that appeal to you, and do not push your body when you are tired. Get adequate rest and exercise. Encourage your body to run on natural energy, not on the false, destructive energy of sugar.

In China, sugar is applied externally to help wounds heal. That's the first genuinely beneficial use for sugar I've ever heard of.

Summing Up

- Avoid sugar in any form: white table sugar, concentrated fruit juice, barley malt, maple syrup, honey, etc. If you use it at all, use it only for special occasions.
- Real all labels and be aware of sugar's many "aliases."
- Chromium picolinate and zinc picolinate help curb sugar cravings.
- Eat at least two meals per day that have significant amounts of protein. This helps keep blood sugar balanced. If you keep your blood sugar balanced, you will never crave sugar again.[36, 37, 38, 39]

CHAPTER 7

Is Alcohol Health-Promoting?

Stay busy, get plenty of exercise, and don't drink too much.
Then again, don't drink too little.
— Herman "Jackrabbit" Smith-Johannsen, at 103

D O UMBRELLAS CAUSE RAIN TO fall? Does rain cause umbrellas to appear? Researchers aren't sure. Some say the number of umbrellas that come out in the rain depends on a signal given by a weather forecaster. Other researchers have found, however, that these numbers do not hold up well in urban environments due to a phenomenon known as the "street side-vendor." Further research is needed.

The human body is complicated. When one thing occurs, like alcohol consumption, and another thing occurs, like health, we cannot say that one caused the other until we understand what causes what. Simultaneous occurrence doesn't mean anything.

Any time we are trying to understand the chain of events responsible for anything from a sports victory to the development of heart disease, many factors have to be taken into consideration, and many can be blown out of proportion. One missed shot at the end of a game may seem to make a team lose, but that one shot did not cause the loss any more than any other missed shot in the game. The player who missed the shot may blame himself for years, yet he is seeing things out of proportion. Any one element in our diet, whether beneficial or detrimental, must be understood in the context of the entire diet. It is the sum total of everything we do in life that keeps us healthy or creates disease.

The residents of Rosetto, Pennsylvania, are well known for their high-fat diet and low rates of heart disease. Their community is very tightly knit, which may in turn have many beneficial health effects. A tight network of social support is a health-building factor that is rarely discussed. It is something that is rare in fragmented societies like America. The drinking of alcohol is often associated with social bonding.

With all of the many factors that affect health, and in particular the health of the heart, can we isolate one food, alcohol, and figure out whether it is beneficial? In countries like France, red wine is credited with keeping heart disease rates lower than those in the United States. There is no question that there are beneficial substances in red wine that protect against cholesterol oxidation and may protect against heart disease. Yet there are also damaging effects from alcohol, which probably lead to the increased rates of cirrhosis of the liver seen in France. And the French rate of heart disease is not as low as it could be. Primitive cultures in which no alcohol is consumed have much lower rates of heart disease than the French.

RED WINE: THE LEAST WORST DRINK

Red wine, not white wine, is loaded with powerful polyphenols that can protect cholesterol from sticking to arteries and causing heart disease. Yet there are many fruits, vegetables, and spices that also pack a wallop of protective power, as well as many vitamin and mineral supplements. So while red wine has unquestionable benefits, the drawbacks suggest you get your protective antioxidants elsewhere.

WHAT IS IT ABOUT RED WINE THAT IS BENEFICIAL?

- It is often drunk in a positive, reinforcing social environment of friends and relatives.
- It is pleasurable and relaxing.
- Copper-containing substances are sprayed on French vineyards. Copper is an important nutrient for the health of the heart and arteries, and copper helps keep cholesterol in normal ranges.
- Red wine contains polyphenols, powerful antioxidants that protect cholesterol from oxidizing.

WHAT IS IT ABOUT ALCOHOL THAT IS DETRIMENTAL?

- Alcohol depletes many nutrients, particularly zinc and magnesium.

- Alcohol can increase the production of free radicals in the body.
- Alcohol can damage the liver.
- Alcohol consumed by pregnant women can lead to low-birth-weight babies with lower IQs.
- Social drinking can progress into alcoholism. Alcoholism is at epidemic levels in America.
- Alcohol damages the brain.
- Alcohol impairs the function of the digestive tract.
- Alcohol may increase the risk of breast cancer.

PROTECTS THEM FROM WHAT?

The French consume large quantities of saturated fat. Red wine is said to protect them from the ill effects of saturated fat. What ill effects?

When researchers see countries like America and Finland, where people eat saturated fats and have high rates of heart disease, they place saturated fat high on their list of offenders. Yet they do not ever look at healthy populations that consume large amounts of saturated fats like the Eskimos, the Masai tribesmen in Africa, and populations in Southeast Asia. If they did, they would realize that heart disease is not caused by saturated fats. Heart disease is caused by nutrient deficiencies, sugar and calorie excess, and free radicals from toxic foods and environmental insults. Saturated fats may get caught in the barroom brawl caused by these factors, but themselves cause nothing. Saturated fats are an essential part of human metabolism. If you ate none, your body would make them.

Garlic

If one were to isolate one food from the French diet that protects against heart disease, it would be garlic. The French eat a lot of garlic, something that has been shown to protect against heart disease in countless ways. In fact, the beneficial side of their alcohol consumption may be its ability to help the body absorb more of the beneficial substances in garlic.

Fruits and Vegetables

The French eat far more fruits and vegetables than Americans, and often eat them raw with all of their valuable antioxidant nutrients intact. Fruits and vegetables are loaded with good things that protect the heart and arteries.

What Other Health-Promoting Things Do the French Do?

Quality of life is very important to the French, and paramount above all else is the quality of food. It must be fresh and full of flavor. Good cooking requires fresh ingredients, and the French do not like processed foods with additives. They like real food, not sugary junk food. They buy fresh produce, meat, and breads daily. They also do not eat between meals as much as Americans do.

French meals are spread over longer periods of time, allowing for better digestion and assimilation of nutrients. Mealtime is often stressful in America. We are, after all, the country that invented the fast-food restaurant. Mealtime in France is a time for relaxing and socializing. And the French do not overeat like Americans do. Their portions are smaller, and their meat is also lower in fat than American meats.

Less Milk

French children are more likely to drink wine with a meal than a glass of milk. They get their calcium from the hundreds of cheeses available in their supermarkets. Xanthine oxidase which is found in homogenized whole milk may be a potent cause of heart disease. Avoiding homogenized whole milk may offer significant benefit.

THE BOTTOM LINE

Optimal nutrition is about isolating the good elements in food and getting more of those. It is also about avoid harmful, toxic substances. Alcohol, even red wine, has some of both. If you want to be optimally healthy, you only want to accentuate the positive. You don't want to set your house on fire and turn on your sprinkler system at the same time.

Don't drink alcohol if you are doing it for health benefits. There are less toxic ways to get the benefits of the antioxidants, polyphenols, and other substances found in red wine. Fruits, vegetables, garlic, spices and herbs, and supplements can give you just as much antioxidant benefit if not more. If you are interested in the protective effects of red wine polyphenols, they are available in supplement form. Alcohol's nutrient-depleting effect is not what a poorly nourished society needs. Its liver-weakening properties are also not needed in a country where the liver is nearly overwhelmed with all of the toxins in our environment.

Can you drink alcohol now and then and be healthy? Yes. An occasional glass of red wine is not going to do that much damage, and does offer some benefits. If it gives you pleasure and is an important part of the way you enjoy life, it may be more unhealthy for you to abstain. Consume red wine or alcohol, however, only after considering its full spectrum of positive and negative effects.

CHAPTER 8

Healthy Cooking Basics

*Cooking is like making love. It should be done with complete
abandon or not at all.*

—Oscar Wilde

A DOPTING HEALTHY COOKING HABITS IS one of the most important things we can do. It increases the amount of nutrients and decreases the toxic substances we ingest. Like
any aspect of maintaining your health, healthy cooking requires principles. You can learn all the facts you want, but if you
don't learn the principles, you will never make it a part of your
life. Facts are forgettable. Principles fit our need to improvise
and make do with the variables of life: the food at hand, the
likes and dislikes of those we live with, and our desire for an
enjoyable, original meal.

We need a new cuisine. The great cuisines of the world
grew up for the most part with little interest in health. When
you step into the kitchen to combine your newfound health-
promoting foods such as whole grains, flaxseed oil, other unrefined oils, expensive organic vegetables, and lower-fat cuts of
meat, you are going up against thousands of years of recipe
development that have accentuated the tastes of fat, sugar, and
white flour.

Learning how to replace these ingredients is crucial for
healthy cooking. Too often, attempts at improving our diet fail
not for any lack of enthusiasm, but because we have been
missing one link in the chain: the ability to make whole foods
taste good. There are many ways to use whole grains, vegetables, unrefined oils, and lower-fat meat and dairy products so
that they are palatable to everyone.

Many of the ways we learned to prepare food are no longer
acceptable. Frying is out. It creates highly toxic products that
destroy the body. Using sugar and white flour is frowned upon

because of the stress these foods place on the body. We get enough salt in our food and do not need to add more. We need, therefore, to look at food preparation in a new way that exploits the natural flavors of food and maximizes their nutritional value. Once you understand and adopt a few simple principles, you will have all you need to begin preparing your food in the healthiest way possible.

SHOULD EVERYTHING BE EATEN RAW?

There are nutritionists who feel we need to eat as many raw foods as possible. This is not a bad idea, because many nutrients can be destroyed in cooking. Yet the nutritional value of foods—even many vegetables—are enhanced by the right amount of cooking. Each food has to be prepared in a way that allows its nutrients to be easily digested.

Not all food can be eaten raw. Foods like beans must be either sprouted or cooked. Meats and fish need to be cooked as well. I know that many people love sushi, but I do not recommend it. Raw fish is a significant source of parasites. Undercooked meats can cause dangerous salmonella and e. coli infections. Soft-boiled and undercooked scrambled eggs can be a source of bad bacteria as well.

Fruits are best eaten raw, but can be baked for a surprisingly sweet dessert. Baked apples and bananas are excellent desserts for children. Fruit can be frozen and put in a blender with half fruit juice and half water for a delicious no-sugar-added shake. Avoid peeling, chopping, or slicing fruits and vegetables until you are ready to serve or cook them.

Vegetables should be eaten raw, steamed, and occasionally stir-fried. Never boil vegetables, for the water will end up with more vitamins than you will. Steaming or cooking vegetables in soups actually helps release more nutrients. Eating a carrot raw will never release as much beta-carotene as juicing, steaming, or cooking it in a soup. Only when the fibers in the plant are broken down can the body absorb its many vitamins and minerals.

Meats, fish, and poultry should be baked, broiled, gas-grilled, and occasionally stir-fried or sautéed. Never fry. Charcoal cooking on the outside grill is, unfortunately, also out. It creates a collection of chemicals that are powerfully carcinogenic. The danger arises from the fat that drips onto the fire and then is changed into a toxic gas that gets redistributed over the meat. The black lines that are burned into the meat are also filled with altered proteins that are poisonous to the body.

Fish such as salmon and sardines are rich in the beneficial omega-3 fats, but the inadequate inspection of seafood has made many wary of fish. Shop from a reputable fish market, and ask how fresh the fish is. Ask if farm-raised fish, such as salmon and catfish, are available. Make sure they come from farms where the water is clean and not filled with antibiotics. Lake fish are more likely to be polluted than those caught in the open ocean. Ask the fish store to allow you to smell a sample of the fish before you buy it. Fish should never smell fishy or have an ammonialike odor. Fresh fish springs back when you touch it and feels firm. Eyes in whole fish should be bright, clear, and unsunken. Cook fish within a matter of hours of buying it, or freeze it for later use. Adding fresh lemon juice or raw garlic to fish before cooking binds toxins that may be present and prevent you from absorbing them.

Fats and oils are perhaps the most important foods to understand and use correctly in cooking. Different cooking temperatures require different oils.

The Right Oil for the Right Temperature
You don't make a twelve-year-old an air traffic controller. Equally out of place are delicate oils in a frying pan. Safflower, sunflower, corn, and walnut oils cannot stand high heat without breaking down into dangerous toxins. When overheated, these polyunsaturated oils may taste good, but they can have devastating effects on your health. You have to know the rules.

Saturated Fats Are Best Able to Handle High Heat. Everyone is trying to eat less saturated fats. Should they be? Saturated fats are those that are solid at room temperature. They are found in foods like meat, butter, dairy products, coconut and palm oils. When saturated fats are not balanced with other nutrients—especially when they are eaten with sugar and without essential fatty acids—they can create disease. Because Americans have made a national sport out of overeating and consuming junk food, the harmful interaction of saturated fats with sugar and white flour has been blamed on saturated fats alone.

Because saturated fat is judged on an uneven playing field, it is thought of as a villain. Instead of using fats that are best designed for high heat-recipes such as saturated fats, we put delicate unsaturated vegetable oils in the deep fryer at McDonald's. They were never made to withstand this heat. No one examined what they would turn into when put under extremely high heat. Not very scientific, and, in the long run, disastrous for our health.

Dangerously high levels of trans fats and other toxic products that come from frying with delicate vegetable oils may take years to do their damage, but the damage they inflict is real. They can cause a wide variety of degenerative diseases. We have enough information now to call for an elimination of delicate oils in all cooking that employs high heat.

You want the right oil for the right cooking job. There are no fats that benefit from heat, so the less you heat fats, the better. When you cook, you don't want to create toxins that kill you. You want to have a tasty meal that doesn't weaken the function of your liver and increase the load of harmful free radicals in the body.

Fats and Oils: Where and How to Use Them			
No-Heat Recipes, Salads	Baking	Sautéing	Stir-Frying
flaxseed, pumpkin-seed, and canola oils, all unrefined vegetable oils	safflower, sesame, corn, and canola oils	sesame oil and high-oleic safflower oil	peanut oil and coconut oil

REPLACING SUGAR

Sugar is one of the most nutrient-depleting substances known. The less we eat, the better. Many recipes contain more sugar than necessary. Amounts recommended can often be decreased by one third to one half and replaced with flour or some other dry ingredient. There are many dishes in which sugar can be omitted completely. Apple pie, for example, can be made without sugar. The sweetness of cooked apples augmented by spices such as cinnamon will satisfy any sweet tooth.

Reduce your use of sugar by adding raisins, dried apricots, or chopped fruit to cereals and cookies. Artificial sweeteners are not recommended, for they perpetuate the need for a highly sweet taste and have caused many negative reactions.

Are There Healthy Sweeteners?

Health food stores sell many products that are sweetened with fruit juice concentrates and other so-called natural sweeteners. While sweeteners such as barley malt, rice syrup, maple syrup, and fructose may have minor benefits over white sugar, they are not much better. They may be used as a transition to getting sugar out of your recipes. They should not be used under the delusion that they are in any way health-promoting.

Always try to include high-fiber foods such as the oatmeal in oatmeal cookies whenever making foods with concentrated sweeteners. While whole-grain, fruit-juice-sweetened cookies cannot be thought of as health foods, they are a vast improvement over the white-flour, white-sugar concoctions sold in supermarkets. They are an acceptable transition food for those moving to a healthier diet.

HERBS AND SPICES

Herbs and spices do more than augment the flavor of food. They offer the body a wide range of immune-boosting substances as well. They are a valuable source of trace minerals and flavonoids—naturally occurring plant pigments with anti-inflammatory and cell-protecting properties. Flavonoids are powerful antioxidants that are many times more powerful than vitamin E, and may soon be thought of as one of the first lines of defense against cancer and heart disease.[40, 41, 42]

Salt use should be limited as much as possible. Salt displaces other minerals such as calcium and increases the risk of stomach cancer. Small amounts may be used to balance other spices. Black pepper is also undesirable for its negative effects on the liver. Try to switch to other herbs and spices.

THE VALUE OF UNREFINED GRAIN PRODUCTS

Grain products when correctly prepared are a valuable source of fiber, vitamins, minerals, and essential fatty acids. Learning how to use grain products effectively, even when they do not comprise a large part of the diet, is an important part of an overall strategy for optimal health.

All Grain Products Should Be:
- Whole and unrefined
- Freshly prepared and responsibly stored
- Organically grown

Whole and Unrefined. When whole-grain flour is turned into white flour, most of its nutritional value is lost. To receive all of the nutritional benefits of grains, they must be in their whole form. "Wheat" bread may look dark and grainy, but if the label does not say "whole wheat," it isn't a whole food. Manufacturers do not like whole-grain products because they go bad quickly and attract pests. These pests are smart enough to reject white flour. We should follow their example.

Freshly Prepared. Turning grains into flours exposes their delicate fats to air. These valuable, fragile fats quickly deteriorate when exposed to oxygen. When these fats spoil, they stress our immune system and are not health-promoting. Whole-grain flours, cut oats, whole cornmeal, and similar products should be purchased through manufacturers who grind their products freshly and keep them refrigerated until they are sold. Otherwise, whole foods such as oatmeal, whole corn grits, and whole-grain flours will lose their benefits and stress your immune system. Flaked oatmeal that has been sitting on supermarket shelves is a good source of fiber but does not offer anywhere near the flavor and benefit of whole oat groats that you buy and flake yourself. The fat in the store-bought flaked oatmeal is in all likelihood rancid as well. Inexpensive, hand-driven oat flakers are available and are highly recommended.

Unrefrigerated whole wheat flour from the supermarket is unacceptable. It has been sitting on the shelf for long periods of time, and is rancid. Even many health food stores unfortunately do not keep their whole-grain flours refrigerated due to the high cost of doing so. Raw wheat germ sold in health food stores is always rancid. You can tell from its bitter taste. Avoid it. The only wheat germ that is fresh is that which is ground in front of you.

Replacing White Flour
Replacing bleached white flour in your cookies and piecrusts is not as difficult as it might seem. Start by mixing white and

whole wheat flour half and half in recipes that call for flour. Better still, switch to the lighter forms of wheat known as spelt and Kamut. Gradually work these into all your favorite recipes. You and your family will enjoy the chewy, nutty taste of these grains. Available in health food stores, these whole grains make excellent cookies, cakes, and piecrusts. Even if you can only make your baking half whole grain, you will significantly increase your fiber, vitamin, and mineral intake.

Eat the "New" Old Grains

Spelt and Kamut are not the only new grains you should try. There are many grains that add more variety to mealtime and increase your intake of valuable nutrients. The more we vary the diet, the better. Not only do we ensure a wider intake of nutrients by doing so, but we lessen the chances of becoming intolerant to a grain by consuming it too often.

- Brown rice comes in many varieties. There is sweet, short-grain rice and aromatic long-grain basmati rice. Experiment with the wide variety of brown rices available at health food and specialty stores. Rice must be organic. Commercial rice is heavily sprayed with pesticides.
- Millet is a grain Americans should get to know. It is wonderful as a side dish or in soups, and tastes like a cross between corn and rice.
- Amaranth is a nutty grain that is high in protein and minerals, and makes a chewy, filling side dish or cereal.
- Whole-grain barley is a rich source of fiber, vitamins, and minerals. Avoid pearled barley, which is refined. Barley has been found to lower cholesterol levels.
- Buckwheat is a grain-like food (really a seed) that is high in fiber and minerals and has a high amount of available protein.
- Quinoa, another grain, offers significant amounts of protein and minerals. Lighter and nuttier in taste than amaranth, it is excellent as a side dish and for recipes such as stuffed peppers.
- Teff is a fascinating, tiny grain from Egypt that has more protein than any other grain.

In the end, incorporating whole foods and the exciting new methods of cooking them into your life will allow you to enjoy food in three different ways. The first is the enjoyment of the full-bodied taste of whole, natural foods. The second is the intellectual appreciation of the many benefits these foods confer through their wide array of nutrients. Thirdly, nutrient-dense foods make you feel good hours after you eat them. Your energy levels remain higher and more stable. By incorporating unrefined, whole foods into your diet, you will be healthier, more energetic, and less likely to develop degenerative diseases that are diet-related.

CHAPTER 9

Top Ten Nutrition Myths

1. **Eating according to the new food pyramid will ensure that you are eating a healthy diet.** Virtually any food can fit into the food pyramid. Ice cream, sugar-laden cookies, fried chips, and refined white flour products. The problem with the food pyramid is that it makes little distinction in food quality. It tells you to minimize fats, but does not tell you which fats are best. It also emphasizes carbohydrates, which for many may be inappropriate.

2. **Eggs should be avoided, for they are high in cholesterol.** Eggs are one of the most nutrient-rich foods known, and there is no evidence that they have any effect on cholesterol levels. They are an excellent source of important nutrients like sulfur, zinc, and choline.

3. **Nuts are fattening.** Nuts have a significant amount of calories, but that does not make them fattening. It is the sum total of the food you eat and the efficiency of your metabolism that will determine whether a food you eat increases your weight. Some actually find nuts an excellent snack to help them curb cravings and lose weight.

4. **You need to exercise to lose weight.** Exercise is an excellent and highly recommended adjunct to the weight loss process, but it is not necessary for healthy and permanent weight loss. Diet and nutrient intake are far more important.

5. **Foods must only be eaten in certain combinations.** There is no research that demonstrates that humans need to eat only certain foods at the same time. Humans are omnivores. Our pancreas secretes fat-, protein-, and carbohydrate-digesting enzymes simultaneously. Throughout history, the human race has thrived on a wide variety of foods eaten in

innumerable combinations. The human body can handle any combination of whole foods eaten at the same time.

6. **Diet and nutrient intake has no effect on arthritis.** Vitamin E, EPA, and glucosamine sulfate are just some of the valuable nutritional aids that have proven effective in helping arthritics. The *Lancet* recently published a study showing the dramatic reduction in pain a vegetarian diet can make. When someone tells you that there is no success with nutritional therapies, check to see who funds that organization. They are often funded by drug companies that make arthritis medications.[43, 44, 45, 46, 47, 48, 49, 50, 51, 52]

7. **Cholesterol-lowering medication will lengthen your life.** Statistics show it will shorten it.

8. **Diets don't work.** Well-designed diets by well-educated nutritionists do, especially when optimal levels of nutrients are included.

9. **There are no magic foods.** Nutrition is science, not magic. If certain foods quench free radicals or protect against cancer, suggesting we eat more of those foods is not a sleight-of-hand trick. It is a well-reasoned suggestion based on solid research, and an important strategy in our fight against degenerative disease. Saying "there are no magic foods" implies that all foods have the same effect on the body. That is ridiculous. Those who downplay the value of superfoods are trying to enforce a brand of mediocre nutrition that has kept Americans dying of degenerative diseases long enough.

10. **Senility is genetic and has little to do with diet.** While there are certainly genetic factors at work in such ailments as Alzheimer's disease and other forms of senility, an overall program of optimal nutrition, including nutrients like niacin and herbs like ginkgo, can play a powerful role in preventing senility and enhancing brain health.

Chapter 10

Top Ten Water Facts

1. **Drink six to eight 8-ounce glasses of water per day.** Pregnant and lactating women and athletes need more. Coffee, tea, and sodas do not count toward your daily water requirement. These drinks act as diuretics and lower the amount of water in your body.

2. **A lack of water can significantly decrease work performance.** It can also cause constipation, and can increase the risk to kidney problems and urinary tract infections.

3. **Don't drink unfiltered tap water.** Chlorine is the most dangerous element in most water supplies. It has been implicated in cancer causation, heart disease, and other health problems. Fluoride may also increase cancer risk. Dr. John Yiamouyiannis's *Fluoride: The Aging Factor* discusses the dangers of fluoride in depth. Other undesirable elements found in tap water include nitrates, radon, lead, and other toxic chemicals. The best forms of water filtration are distillation, or a reverse osmosis filter combined with a solid carbon filter. If there is no fluoride added to your water, then a solid carbon filter alone will suffice. Taste is no indication of water's safety. Make sure to get a filter for your shower. Taking a shower in chlorinated water is as bad as drinking it.

4. **Highly sweetened drinks are not absorbed and used by the body as quickly as plain water.** Cold water, between 40 to 50 degrees Fahrenheit, is absorbed best.

5. **Drink water regularly throughout the day.** Don't wait until you are thirsty to replenish your body's water supply.

6. **Fresh fruits and vegetables contain a lot of water.** People who eat a lot of fresh fruits and vegetables can drink less water.

7. **Switching to a diet higher in fiber increases your need for water.**

8. **Athletes should not consume high-fiber foods such as whole grains, whole grain cereals, or apples right before exercise,** as high-fiber foods can pull water from the body into the intestinal tract.

9. **Older Americans have decreased thirst** and need to pay special attention to drinking enough water.

10. **Drinking more water does not increase your tendency to bloat.** In fact, drinking water will decrease bloating. Salt and sodium-rich foods, imbalanced female hormones, and poor cardiac function are the most common causes for bloating.

CHAPTER 11

Top Ten Things to Put on Your Shopping List

1. **Fresh fruits and vegetables,** organic if possible. Fresh produce has more nutrients per calorie than any other food. They should be juiced, eaten raw, or lightly steamed.

2. **Fermented dairy products** like yogurt. Buy plain, sugar-free varieties that are free of artificial sweeteners. Add your own fruit for flavor.

3. **Organic virgin flaxseed, canola, or olive oil.**

4. **Spring or distilled water** if you do not have a high-quality water filter in your house. Don't buy bottled filtered tap water. Read labels.

5. **Dried beans, lentils, and black-eyed peas.** Precooked varieties may also be used for convenience.

6. **Raw nuts,** especially almonds, walnuts, hazelnuts, and brazil nuts still in their shell. Avoid raw peanuts. Organic nuts are best.

7. **Whole-grain pastas, breads, and snacks.** If it doesn't say "whole" on the ingredient listing, as in "whole wheat flour" or "whole durham flour," it isn't.

8. **Unfermented green tea,** Cafix, Celestial Seasonings' "Iced Delight," or any other natural herbal drink mix that does not contain sugar or artificial sweeteners.

9. **Salsa,** mild or spicy, as a replacement for sugar-laden ketchup.

10. **Herbs and spices,** including garlic, ginger, thyme, rosemary, basil, cayenne pepper, and turmeric.

PART II

Supplements

CHAPTER 12

Are Supplements Necessary?

Evidence indicates that the bulk of illness in modern societies is the result of an unrecognized disease cluster I call "modernization disease syndrome." This cluster is caused by a multitude of food and dietary modifications interacting metabolically with stress and exercise deficiency. The food modifications have never been tested for their collective safety by health authorities, and it seems clear they interact in the body to produce a new kind of deadly synergistic malnutrition that is not caused by any one factor alone. . . . These disturbances, when playing against genetic variations, can cause just about every illness known to medicine.

—Donald Rudin, M.D., The Omega-3 Phenomenon

A S YOU SIT ON AN airplane as it waits at the gate before takeoff, the captain enters the passenger section. He has a special request. He has flown this plane innumerable times and would like to know if anyone would mind if he took a wing flap off as a memento. All raise their hands.

If only we had the same regard for our bodies. We fly through life with many missing parts—vitamins, minerals, and essential fatty acids—and have little concern about what may result.

We have nothing to justify our complacency. No study of the American diet has ever shown that we get all the vitamins and minerals we need for optimal health through food. Every study reveals deficiencies or suboptimal intakes of many micronutrients. This is a large part of the reason why we have so much heart disease, cancer, osteoporosis, and other life-shortening degenerative diseases.

Diet- and nutrient-deficiency-related degenerative diseases kill more Americans than anything else. Bathing our cells in a nutritionally opulent environment through an optimal diet and the judicious use of supplements can significantly reduce

79

this risk. Without optimal nutrient intake, we cannot expect to live a healthy life in a toxic world filled with processed, nutrient-poor foods.

To Supplement or Not to Supplement

Dietitians, the largest group of nutritionists in America, say that we don't need to supplement, yet a recent survey showed two-thirds of all dietitians take supplements. Cardiologists do not recommend supplements to their patients, yet two-thirds of them take antioxidants to protect their own hearts and arteries.[53] The cover story of the March 1987 issue of *Consumer Reports* featured an article called "The Vitamin Pushers." It declared supplements unnecessary. In the back of the same issue, you could order *The Consumer Reports Guide to Vitamin and Mineral Supplements.* Who's fooling whom?

Crayhon's Law of Nutritional Supplements:

Those Who Say We Do Not Need Supplements Should Not Be Allowed to Take Them

Countless studies show Americans do not consume even RDA levels of B_6, folic acid, magnesium, and zinc. This is especially true with the young and elderly. The refined flours, refined oils, and canned and fried foods that make up much of the American diet not only do not contain enough vitamins and minerals to meet the RDA, they deplete us of the vitamins and minerals we consume. Fruits and vegetables lose many vitamins on their long voyage from the farm to your table, and lack minerals due to overfarmed soils. Don't be deceived into thinking that you can get optimal amounts of vitamins and minerals through food. There isn't a single scientific study to prove that it can be done.

Supplements are extraordinarily safe. According to the National Center for Health Statistics, 125,000 people died in 1992 as a direct result of drugs prescribed by doctors, while 9,000 people died in 1992 as a result of food poisoning. No one died that year due to the use of vitamin or mineral supplements.

Some say supplements are a waste of money. Americans spend more money on potato chips than they do on vitamins.

Potato chips are filled with trans fats that cause disease. The soda industry dwarfs the vitamin industry, and, even in the most conservative circles, sugar is recognized for promoting dental caries, obesity, and heart disease, and raising triglycerides. If we are trying to get Americans healthier, why don't we go after the empty-calorie toxic foods that create disease, like sugar and trans fats, instead of supplements, which do much to prevent it?

Many people say that they don't like taking optimal doses of nutrients through supplements because they don't think they are "natural." That is like complaining, "Do I really have to go to the bank every week and pick up the dividend check on my trust fund? It's more natural to work for the money." We ought to be glad that the most valuable elements in food have been isolated. They are conveniently within our reach so we can have them in optimal amounts instead of relying on the small quantities supplied by food. Taking supplements is not natural. Taking supplements is *optimal.*

Some say that we shouldn't take supplements because we didn't have them in Stone Age times. Where did we get this idealistic picture of prehistoric life? "The Flintstones"? Few would benefit from supplements more than Paleolithic mankind. Their lives were short and stressful. They had a very irregular food supply that changed with the seasons and fluctuations in animal populations. Everyone, no matter which millennium they hail from, could have benefited from supplements.

The soils in Egypt and Iran are devoid of zinc due to thousands of years of farming. Our soils are becoming similarly depleted. Our body needs trace minerals like chromium and selenium that are poorly supplied by our soils. If we do not get them through supplements, we are going to be deficient and develop a degenerative disease.

The "get everything from the diet" routine just doesn't work in the modern world for the following reasons:

- Even an optimal selection of foods does not give us enough antioxidants to defend ourselves against toxic outgassing from office equipment, cigarette smoke, smog, and alcohol.
- The average person is exposed to more than five hundred chemicals in the home environment and seven hundred chemicals in drinking water that are known to deplete many nutrients.[54]

- Soils are depleted of minerals due to chemical farming methods, acid rain, overfarming, and topsoil erosion.
- Ninety percent of us are deficient in chromium, an essential trace mineral poorly supplied by the American diet.
- Eighty percent of the carbohydrates consumed by Americans are in the form of refined flours and sugars, which are very poor sources of B_6, folic acid, pantothenic acid, zinc, and manganese essential for health.
- The 133 pounds of sugar Americans eat each year depletes B vitamins and minerals.
- Only 9% of the population eats the recommended five servings of vitamin-rich fruits and vegetables.
- Americans eat 230 more calories per day than they did fifteen years ago. Our diet consists of refined foods. Increasing our consumption of nutrient-depleted foods means we have an even higher requirement for the vitamins and minerals needed to metabolize them.
- Those who exercise regularly have a much higher need for antioxidants and minerals.
- Vitamin B_2 is needed by those with hypothyroid in amounts greater than can be found in food.[55]
- Men and women need to be optimally nourished long before they have children.
- More than 10% of calories consumed in America come from alcoholic beverages. Alcohol depletes B vitamins, zinc, and magnesium.[56]
- Our epidemic of degenerative diseases is caused by multiple nutrient deficiencies.
- Prescription and over-the-counter medications can deplete nutrients and create deficiencies.
- Birth control pills create B_6 deficiencies and increase the need for B_6 beyond what the diet can supply.
- Illness increases our need for vitamin C and zinc well beyond what food can supply.
- Millions of Americans are dieting and need supplements just to meet minimal nutrient requirements. Dieting increases free radical production, and optimal levels of antioxidants are needed to reduce damage to the liver and other organs that can occur during weight loss.

If your physician tells you he does not believe in vitamins, tell him that you don't have to believe in them. You just have to take them.

THE RDAs

The RDAs were not established to help you achieve optimal health. They are merely:

- Amounts of nutrients needed to prevent deficiency plus a safety factor of two to three.
- Amounts needed by populations, not individuals.
- Amounts of nutrients for those who digest and metabolize food normally.
- Amounts for healthy persons, not for those who are sick.

The RDAs were never designed to prevent heart disease or cancer, or encourage optimal health. They are designed to do little more than prevent deficiency. The amount of vitamin C that prevents scurvy is 10 milligrams per day. The amount that helps prevent heart disease is at least thirty times that.

The lack of value of the RDAs is underscored by the fact that for many nutrients there is little more than a cursory examination of the population's intake before an allowance is determined. Example: vitamin E. Because the body can recycle small amounts of vitamin E, acute deficiency is rare. The RDA was set at the amount that most Americans were eating because the people examined seemed to be healthy. No matter that nearly half these Americans would die of heart disease that is caused or aggravated by a lack of optimal levels of vitamin E. At the moment they were looked at, they appeared fine.

What does the RDA mean to you and me? Minimum wage nutrition.

You can't change the RDA without causing a tremendous ripple effect. If someone were to admit that optimal levels of nutrients are needed and cannot be supplied by food, a tidal wave of revisionist nutritional and medical thinking would be needed that would force many scientists and institutions to admit they were wrong. For now, such thinking is forbidden in politically correct medical and nutrition circles. The health of the nation and our ability to fight off an onslaught of increasing degenerative diseases is at stake. If we do not embrace the overwhelming findings that support optimal nutrition, the health of the nation will only decline further.

The RDA does not need to be improved. It needs to be replaced. And in the meantime, its very limited meaning should remove it from any prescriptions for individual needs. Nutritional thinking and the health of the population will not change until we understand that we need much more optimal levels of nutrients. The best solution is an individual daily allowance (ODA) that will cover all of our vitamin and mineral needs abundantly. The ODA is outlined in Shari Lieberman's readable and highly recommended book, *The Real Vitamin and Mineral Book.*

The need for supplements for disease prevention is so well documented that those who do not take at least conservative doses of antioxidants should be thought of as reckless. They are allowing their bodies to undergo damage that is unnecessary. Even doses as small as 500 milligrams of vitamin C, 100 IUs (international units) of vitamin E, 100 micrograms of selenium, and 25 milligrams of zinc can make a significant difference in long-term health. Insurance companies will one day lower rates for those who take optimal levels of nutrients. They may even start to give them away for free as an incentive.

PHYTOCHEMICALS

New beneficial substances are constantly being discovered in the vegetable kingdom called *phytochemicals*. There is no question that we should eat plenty of produce. Researchers who say we can't get these substances through supplements, however, are not correct. Supplements of many of these beneficial compounds *are* available. Secondly, statements like "You can't get these phytochemicals through supplements" imply that supplements are inferior to food. You may not be able to get all the beneficial compounds found in produce with a pill, and no one suggests you try. But food will never give you the optimal amounts of vitamin C, vitamin E, and trace minerals you need. Eat plenty of vegetables. But don't forget your vitamin C and E. You can't get their full protective effect through the amounts found in food no matter how well you eat.

Many people say that we should eat a better diet instead of taking supplements, as if it were impossible to do both at the same time. Those who supplement with vitamins and minerals are not predominantly junk food addicts. They are often people who care about their health and want to do everything they can to augment it. Cleaning up your diet is good. Taking supplements is good. Do both.

Many people are reluctant to replace their onion rings with a salad. It is very difficult to get children, men, and the elderly in particular to change their diet. It can be easy to get them to take supplements. Most people could benefit from improving their diets and should do so. But let's not discourage those who eat junk food diets from using supplements. They need them more than anyone.

WHO CAN PROVE THAT FOOD IS ENOUGH?

Question those who tell you that food alone can satisfy your nutritional needs. Ask them for a study that can prove their point. There are none. It is a very dangerous deception to masquerade such beliefs as scientifically valid. If believed, such information will deprive you of optimal health.

Expensive Urine?
People often claim that supplements are not needed and merely create expensive urine. Giving your body a wide selection of supplements is inviting it to a smorgasbord of beneficial nutrients. It takes what it wants and excretes the rest. So long as care is exercised to avoid excessive iron and vitamins A and D, and an intelligent supplemental strategy is employed, an abundant intake of beneficial nutrients is remarkably health-promoting. For the vast majority of nutrients, it is far better to err on the side of luxury and allow your body an abundant supply than to let suboptimal deficiencies develop.

Nutrients in the urine are good. They are a sign that the body has so many nutrients, it can afford to give some away. Don't let anyone give you the unproven argument that vitamins cause kidney stones. Recent studies confirm vitamin C does not cause kidney stones. Vitamin B_6 and magnesium actually prevent kidney stones. A lack of these two nutrients along with a high-sugar, low-fiber diet is the real cause.[57, 58, 59, 60, 61]

A nutrient that all of us consume that always goes out in the urine is water. As water supplies decrease in states like California, people may be told to drink less water because they are just making expensive urine. Water plays many valuable roles in promoting health as it travels through the body. Most of us do not drink enough. It is not merely going through us; it is promoting our health. The same is true with all other essential nutrients.

I want expensive urine. I want an expensive heart, brain, arteries, glands, and bloodstream, too. I want every part of my body expensive if this means optimally nourished. This costs me $300 per year, less than a dollar a day. The return on my investment has been and will be a much happier, healthier, and more productive life.

CHAPTER 13

B Complex Vitamins

They are going to make vitamins illegal. I guess the new saying will be "Just Say No to Riboflavin."

—Conan O'Brian

TWO KINDS OF VITAMINS

Just as there are cars for land and boats for sea, there are different classes of vitamins for the two types of bodily terrain. There are watery nutrients for blood and other fluids—vitamin C and the B complex—and there are fat-soluble vitamins like beta-carotene and vitamins A, D, E, and K for fatty tissues. Optimal amounts of both kinds are necessary for high-level wellness and disease prevention. Let's begin our examination of vitamins by looking at the water-soluble B complex.

B Complex Vitamins

The B complex is an important group of nutrients the body must acquire through the diet or from the intestinal flora in order to transform food into energy, maintain a strong immune system, balance many of the body's hormones, and perform a variety of other tasks. Each of the B vitamins has individual characteristics. While it is often best to take them as a complex, there are times when taking them individually will yield a greater therapeutic benefit.

It is important to get optimal amounts of B vitamins. Sugar, white flour, alcohol, stress, and environmental pollution can deplete them. Signs of marginal B vitamin deficiency can be difficult to detect. It is far better to get an optimal intake of Bs than risk the nervous system deterioration and other problems associated with low intake of these vitamins. Since only 20% of the carbohydrates consumed in America are from whole-grain sources that are rich in B vitamins, supplementation is recommended.

B₁ or Thiamine. Vitamin B_1 is essential for the health of the nervous system and for the breakdown of food into energy. Subclinical deficiencies of B_1 can lead to lower energy levels. A frank deficiency of vitamin B_1 is associated with aggressive behavior and other personality changes. Vitamin B_1 deficiency is common in alcoholics and schizophrenics. Up to 30% of those who enter psychiatric wards have been found to be deficient in thiamine.[62]

B_1 has been shown to be deficient in those with Alzheimer's disease.[63] This is an indication that long-term subclinical deficiency of B_1 may cause deterioration of the brain.[64] B_1 deficiency can also lead to heart failure and damage the nervous system.[65]

B_1 is an important nutrient for diabetics. It protects against the development of diabetic neuropathy, a complication of diabetes that results in nerve damage.[66]

Food sources for B_1 include all whole grains, meats, fish, poultry, legumes, nuts, and seeds.

B₁ Guidelines

- B_1 is important for energy production, detoxification, heart function, and the health of the nervous system.
- The need for B_1 increases as an increased amounts of calories, particularly starches and sugars, are consumed.
- Supplemental doses of B_1 can range between 10 and 500 milligrams per day. For most people 10–50 milligrams per day will supply optimal amounts.

B₂ or Riboflavin. Vitamin B_2 is another nutrient that helps us release the energy in food. Without B_2, vitamin B_6 cannot be used by the body. Supplements of B_2 have been used at doses of 25 milligrams per day to increase the effectiveness of B_6.[67]

Riboflavin is a protective nutrient through its critical role in activating the powerful antioxidant glutathione. B_2 allows the body to reuse glutathione in its battle against toxic chemicals and free radicals.[68] People with cataracts, diabetes, and malaria need to ensure that they have optimal amounts of B_2 so that their antioxidant and immune systems will function optimally.

Eyes that are sensitive to light may be a sign of riboflavin deficiency. Skin disorders, particularly around the lips and nose, as well as cracks around the corners of the mouth, are also signs of deficiency.[69, 70]

Food sources for B_2 include dairy products, whole grains, meats, seafood, nuts, seeds, and legumes.

B_2 Guidelines

- B_2 is needed for energy production, growth, healthy eyes and skin, and the production of red blood cells.
- B_2 regenerates one of the body's great protectors, glutathione.
- Optimal supplemental doses range between 10 and 100 milligrams per day.

Vitamin B_3. Vitamin B_3 comes in two forms: niacin and niacinamide. While the body's need for vitamin B_3 can be satisfied by either, these two different kinds of vitamin B_3 have different effects when used at amounts higher than those supplied by food.

Niacin. Niacin is an effective cholesterol-lowering agent. Niacin has also been used by Dr. Abram Hoffer in treatment of schizophrenia, and may also prevent senility through its ability to stimulate circulation. Doses of 100 milligrams per day may be adequate for this preventive effect. Doses of more than 50 milligrams can initially lead to a harmless but annoying flushing reaction that turns skin red, but this reaction will discontinue if niacin is taken regularly.

Niacin has been used for over forty years as one of the most effective ways of lowering LDL cholesterol and triglycerides.[71, 72, 73, 74] Niacin also raises beneficial HDL cholesterol by 31%.[75] This is a highly significant finding. HDL is very protective against heart disease. Taking a dose of 100 milligrams and increasing gradually to 1 gram (1,000 milligrams) per day is well tolerated and has been shown to lower total cholesterol and raise HDL levels.[76, 77] Niacin has also been shown to reduce the incidence of nonfatal heart attacks and increase the long-term survival of victims of heart attacks.[78]

Niacin may not be the first supplement of choice for diabetics interested in lowering their blood cholesterol levels. Thirteen diabetic patients given 4.5 grams of niacin in divided doses had their cholesterol and triglyceride levels lowered effectively, but blood sugar levels increased 16%—not a desirable result.[79] Low-dose niacin combined with chromium has been found to be as effective at lowering cholesterol as high-dose niacin alone. This for many would seem to be the better choice, especially for diabetics, since chromium normalizes blood sugar as well.[80]

Inositol Hexanicotinate: No-Flush Niacin. Inositol hexanicotinate is the only form of time-released niacin that is recommended. It does not produce a flushing reaction and is very well tolerated by the body. It may be the best form for cholesterol lowering. Other time-released forms of niacin are not recommended. Even in low doses, they can irritate the liver.[81, 82, 83]

Although niacin is extraordinarily safe, when used in high doses it should be taken with the guidance of a health-care practitioner.

Niacinamide. Niacinamide, the other form of vitamin B_3, will not cause flushing, nor will it lower cholesterol or improve circulation. Yet it has a range of other benefits. It was used in the 1940s to reduce the insulin requirements of diabetics. Many studies have shown that niacinamide protects the beta cells of the pancreas from damage that leads to Type I insulin-dependent diabetes. Doses of 100 to 500 milligrams per day seem to offer the most benefit, and are completely safe.[84]

In a two-and-a-half-year study of eighty thousand New Zealanders aged five to seven years old, niacinamide significantly reduced the incidence of diabetes. The twenty thousand treated with niacinamide developed only four cases of diabetes, while the sixty thousand who were not given B_3 developed fifty-two cases. Niacinamide therefore afforded a 75% reduction in the occurrence of this incurable disease. Though this is a preliminary study, it indicates that this inexpensive, nontoxic nutrient may offer unique benefit to anyone with a family history of diabetes.

Niacinamide has been found to be a very effective treatment for osteoarthritis. Dr. Kaufman was a physician who did extensive research in the 1940s with this form of vitamin B_3. He found that doses between 500 milligrams and 3 grams per day were a very valuable treatment for osteoarthritis. Using more than 500 milligrams of niacinamide per day is best done under the supervision of a health professional.

Food sources for vitamin B_3, usually in the form of niacinamide, are meat, poultry, dairy products, seafood, nuts, and seeds.

Vitamin B_3 Guidelines
- B_3 requirements can be met through either niacin or niacinamide.
- Niacin lowers cholesterol, and no-flush niacin (inositol hexanicotinate) is the best and safest form.
- Regular crystalline niacin in doses of over 50 milligrams may cause uncomfortable but harmless flushing.
- Niacinamide has been found helpful for osteoarthritis.
- Niacin is the more beneficial form, though some may find the initial flushing annoying. Optimal amounts of niacin will differ, but range between 50 and 200 milligrams per day, more for therapeutic purposes.

Folic Acid. Folic acid is named after the green leafy foliage that is the richest source for this nutrient. Folic acid is needed for the health of gums, red blood cells, skin, and gastrointestinal tract. It prevents birth defects, cancer, and heart disease, and is important for a strong immune system. It may also be helpful in the treatment in certain forms of mental illness. Most Americans do not consume even half of the RDA for folic acid.[85] Because of this vitamin's importance, those who do not eat abundant amounts of fresh vegetables each day should supplement. The operative word here is *fresh*, because folic acid is easily lost from vegetables through cooking and exposure to light. A great deal of folic acid is lost the first day the vegetables are picked, put on a truck, and taken to market. Fresh vegetables you pick and eat immediately are the richest source for this fragile B vitamin. Folic acid's importance and our low intake of it are both so well recognized that folic acid fortification of grain products is now being proposed.

Women who are pregnant or trying to become pregnant must ensure that their multivitamin contains at least 800 micrograms of folic acid. The healthy development of the nervous system in the first weeks of an embryo's life depends on adequate folic acid along with other key nutrients such as zinc, pantothenic acid, and essential fatty acids found in flaxseed oil.

Optimal intake of folic acid also plays a role in the prevention of heart disease. Optimal levels of folic acid and B_6 both keep homocysteine—a dangerous substance that can cause significant damage to arteries—from elevating to damaging levels. Many researchers believe that increasing your intake of folic acid and B_6 is one of the keys to decreasing the risk of a heart attack. The amount of these nutrients found even in a healthful diet may not be enough to lower homocysteine in everyone.[86]

Food sources for folic acid include dark leafy greens, whole grains, broccoli, beets, asparagus, and citrus fruits.

Folic Acid Guidelines
- Eat plenty of fresh fruits and vegetables and take a multivitamin that has at least 400 micrograms of folic acid.
- Pregnant women should take at least 800 micrograms but not more than 3,000 micrograms of folic acid per day, ideally for many months before conception.
- Make sure to take B_{12} along with folic acid, as folic acid can mask signs of B_{12} deficiency.
- Most should try to get at least 400 micrograms per day in a multivitamin. Pregnant women need at least 800 micrograms.

Pantothenic Acid. Pantothenic acid, previously known as vitamin B_5, is needed for the body to burn food, for optimal energy levels, and for wound healing. Pantothenic acid is necessary for the manufacture of adrenal hormones, and has been found to be an important supplement for those who are under stress. Many studies demonstrate pantethine, the activated form of pantothenic acid, can effectively lower blood triglyceride and cholesterol levels.[87, 88, 89]

Supplement with at least 100 milligrams per day of pantothenic acid if you have rheumatoid arthritis, duodenal ulcers, or if you are about to undergo any form of surgery. Pantothenic acid in optimal amounts has been found to help accelerate would healing.[90] It is also important for maintaining a strong immune defense.[91]

Food sources include whole grains, milk, eggs, and milk. The bacteria of the intestinal tract also make pantothenic acid. Refined foods and grain products have very little pantothenic acid.

Pantothenic Acid Guidelines
- Try to get at least 100 milligrams per day in a high-quality multivitamin.
- Optimal doses for those under stress or with joint inflammation range up to 1,000 milligrams.

Vitamin B_6 or Pyridoxine. Vitamin B_6 is needed for brain function, the growth of red blood cells, skin health, immune function, and for the prevention and treatment of a wide range of degenerative diseases.

Adequate B_6 is needed for optimal immune function. It is needed in supplemental amounts by those who are ill. One study found that vitamin B_6 was deficient in a group of AIDS patients despite the fact that they were consuming adequate amounts of B_6 in their diet. Thirty percent of the group were deficient while another 34% were marginally deficient. This lack of B_6 was correlated with a decrease in immune function in these patients.[92, 93]

B_6 has also been found helpful in the nutritional support of asthma and PMS. It is has also been found to be a natural diuretic. Those on oral contraceptives develop mild deficiencies and also require high levels of B_6. B_6 has been shown to help normalize blood pressure. It is also important for athletes and can be depleted by vigorous exercise.

B_6 is needed for the metabolism of protein, and should be used as a supplement whenever higher levels of protein are consumed. B_6 also helps alleviate the symptoms of monosodium glutamate sensitivity. Those sensitive to MSG should supplement with at least 50 milligrams of B_1, B_2, and B_6 daily, especially if they consume significant amounts of processed foods.

It is believed that 30%–40% of the population may have trouble converting B_6 to one of its main active forms in the body, P5P (pyridoxyl-5-phosphate).[94] For such persons, it may be extremely important to use this activated form of B_6 or the benefits of B_6 may not be seen. The body does not activate B_6 effectively in many disease states.[95, 96]

Vitamin B_6 has been found to help decrease the nausea associated with pregnancy in doses as low as 75 milligrams per day. It has no side effects on the mother or fetus at this dose.[97]

Dr. Leo Galland has found that two thirds of those who suffer from an overgrowth of the yeast candida albicans have altered vitamin B_6 metabolism. The presence of candida prevents B_6 from being metabolized into its active P5P form. This may in turn be due to a deficiency of zinc, magnesium, and B_2, all of which are required for adequate B_6 activation. For candida sufferers, P5P may be an essential supplement until zinc, magnesium, and B_2 levels return to normal.[98, 99]

B_6 and magnesium are helpful for a subset of autistic children. Although only 15% to 30% of the children studied show improvement on magnesium and B_6, the improvements in auditory-evoked responses were significant.[100]

B_6 has been shown to reduce the pain of carpal tunnel syndrome, a debilitating condition caused by the compression of the median nerve in the wrist. Twenty CTS adults who were given 200 milligrams of B_6 per day all showed significant decrease in pain after three months of supplementation. Those with CTS who do not respond to B_6 after a period of months should try the activated form of vitamin B_6, pyridoxyl-5-phosphate (P5P).[101] Many studies have confirmed the benefits of B_6 for CTS, suggesting that a course of B_6 be tried before resorting to surgery.

B_6 has been reported to cause a reversible numbness in those taking more than 1,000 milligrams per day of B_6. The people who took these large doses did not balance them with correspondingly high amounts of other B vitamins, which should always be done when taking higher amounts of any one of the Bs. Secondly, there is rarely any benefit from B_6 above 200 milligrams per day when taken as a supplement, and doses up to this amount are completely safe and without side effects.

Food sources for B_6 include whole grains, bananas, nuts, meat, fish, poultry, and legumes.

B_6 Guidelines

- If you take more than 100 milligrams of B_6 per day, balance it with correspondingly higher intakes of other members of the B complex.
- Make sure you are getting 300 milligrams of magnesium per day and at least 10 milligrams of B_2 per day to ensure that you metabolize B_6 correctly.
- If you are using B_6 for therapeutic purposes, such as for PMS, bloating, or carpal tunnel syndrome, take it at a different meal than the rest of the B complex.
- The activated form of B_6 is called pyridoxyl-5-phosphate (P5P). If you do not derive therapeutic benefit from B_6

(called pyridoxine HCL on vitamin labels), you may find P5P helpful.

- For heart disease prevention and general health, 50 milligram one to two times per day should suffice for most people.

Vitamin B_{12}. Vitamin B_{12} is found in animal products, and is a crucial nutrient for the health of the nervous system and the development of red blood cells. Although it may take years to develop a B_{12} deficiency, negative effects on mental function and other areas of bodily function can occur before anemia and other clear signs of B_{12} deficiency develop.

It is difficult to determine when a person needs supplemental vitamin B_{12}. Even if many of the available tests show adequate B_{12} status, there may be nothing better than symptoms in certain cases to judge the need for B_{12}. Signs of B_{12} deficiency are dementia and depression. Deficiency symptoms also include paleness and numbness and tingling in the toes and fingers. Many patients who have shown normal levels of B_{12} in standard tests have shown clinical benefit from vitamin B_{12} injections. Blood levels in those who are deficient in B_{12} can be normal up to 30% of the time. Because of the dangers involved in being B_{12} deficient, it is wiser to err on the side of caution and supplement with B_{12}, or, more optimally, receive injections from a physician when even the possibility of benefit from B_{12} exists.

Supplementing with vitamin B_{12} may be very important for the long-term health of those who eat no animal products at all.[102] Lack of B_{12}, which may occur in the elderly and strict vegetarians—vegans and macrobiotic devotees—can cause slowly progressing and irreversible nerve damage.[103, 104]

Pernicious anemia is the anemia that results when the body has low levels of vitamin B_{12}. It is the classic sign of B_{12} insufficiency. Yet new evidence suggests that B_{12} can be deficient even in the absence of anemia. Even in instances when the blood does not indicate it, B_{12} may be dangerously deficient and can contribute to such problems as mental deterioration, confusion, depression, and other cognitive problems.[105, 106]

Oral B_{12} has been found to be an effective treatment for pernicious anemia when B_{12} is taken in the range of 300 to 1,000 micrograms per day.[107] Doses of 5 to 20 micrograms are ineffective for this problem—another instance in which RDA levels are not enough. Doses of 1,000 micrograms of B_{12} have been tolerated well with no adverse side effects. When pernicious anemia is present, avoid the use of high-dose folic acid supplements unless you also take significant amounts of B_{12}. Folic acid alone will remove the blood symptoms of pernicious anemia, but will not stop the nerve damage caused by B_{12} deficiency. It is because of the chance that folic acid might mask a B_{12} deficiency that supplements of folic acid are limited to a maximum dose of 800 micrograms per tablet. A better solution would be to require B_{12} to be added to all high dose folic acid supplements.[108, 109]

B_{12} shots have also been found very effective in helping bursitis, regardless of whether or not there is a B_{12} deficiency. Researchers and physicians have found that there are many cases in which B_{12} injections or supplementation should not be withheld merely because B_{12} levels are normal. B_{12} supplementation is extraordinarily safe. The only danger of B_{12} is not getting enough.[110]

Virtually all animal products contain vitamin B_{12}, and virtually all plant products contain none. B_{12} is found, however, in fortified cereals and B_{12}-fortified soy milk. Strict vegetarians in India would probably not want to know that the small amount of dead insects in their grain products keeps them from developing a B_{12} deficiency.

B_{12} Guidelines
- If you are a vegan, follow a macrobiotic diet, or for any reason avoid all animal and dairy products, supplement regularly with at least 500 micrograms of B_{12}.
- If you suffer from any form of mental deterioration, seek medical care immediately. Even if there are no test results indicating a B_{12} deficiency, increase your intake of all of the B vitamins. Talk to your physician about B_{12} injections.
- The preferred supplemental form of B_{12} is hydroxycobalamin.
- Most people who eat animal products and have healthy digestion do not require B_{12} supplements.

CHAPTER 14

Vitamin C

VITAMIN C OR ASCORBIC ACID

Vitamin C has the widest range of applications in both the prevention and treatment of disease of any nutrient ever studied. It has, at the same time, demonstrated an extraordinarily wide range of safety. For this reason, vitamin C is one of the most widely supplemented vitamins throughout the world. It is one of the most important antioxidant and immune-enhancing nutrients needed by the human body. The research demonstrating the benefits of vitamin C could fill a small library. If vitamin C were a drug, it would have more benefit and safety than any other drug we now possess.

Many studies have shown vitamin C to be one of the premier antioxidant nutrients in the body. By preventing much of the damaging effects of free radicals, vitamin C plays an important preventive role in virtually all degenerative diseases. Vitamin C is also very important for protecting the cells of the immune system so they can defend the body more effectively. Vitamin C is also needed for healthy gums, skin, and the connective tissue that holds the body together. Vitamin C also protects vitamins B_1, B_2, B_5, folic acid and vitamins A and E from deteriorating in the body.

Did Our Livers Once Make Vitamin C?
Our livers have three enzymes that do absolutely nothing. Their only function would be to turn glucose into vitamin C. If only our liver weren't missing the fourth enzyme needed to make this transformation, our bodies would be able to make vitamin C. This has led many scientists to believe that our

livers once made vitamin C in multigram doses as most mammals do. The goat, for example, can make 17 grams per day of vitamin C. Recent research shows that the gene responsible for the inactive enzyme has undergone significant mutation. It appears obvious that at one point in human history we made our own vitamin C.[111] Combine this with the fact that our ancestral diet had between 400 milligrams and 2 grams of vitamin C per day, and you can see that the RDA of 60 milligrams per day is completely inadequate.

One of the reasons why vitamin C may suffice in small amounts when we are healthy is that when normal conditions exist, the body's cells are capable of recycling some of the vitamin C that it uses up. This is why smaller doses in healthy individuals can suffice without creating signs of severe deficiency, the only thing that scientists who establish the RDA look for. But for those who are experiencing an inflammatory illness, stress, heavy metal intoxication, or a disease of any kind, the body cannot recycle vitamin C to meet the increased needs. It is one thing to have a shotgun if you are defending yourself against a single wild animal and you have time to reload. It's quite another if you have to defend yourself against a stampeding herd. You don't have the luxury of time to regenerate vitamin C at a leisurely pace. It's like trying to put out a building fire with a garden hose. Normal amounts of vitamin C in acute illness are not going to make much of a difference. They cannot handle the torrential downpour of free radicals.

No one would look for vitamin C in the minimal dosage range to perform the complete eradication of free radicals that can only be, in most instances, accomplished with supplements. No one should expect one glass of orange juice to supply all of the vitamin C needed to offer optimal protection against heart disease and cancer.

Because there are really two applications of vitamin C with two different effects, we should think of vitamin C as two different substances:

Vitamin C_1:Doses of vitamin C up to 100 milligrams per day. This amount will protect only against scurvy and ailments related to acute vitamin C deficiency.

Vitamin C_2:Oral and intravenous doses of vitamin C from 100 milligrams to 100 grams per day and beyond. These amounts neutralize free radicals, prevent degenerative diseases, and boost the immune system.

Only by understanding the two different effects of vitamin C in different dosage ranges will we end the outdated argument that high doses are merely excreted in the urine. Vitamin C in these two different dosage ranges offer completely different benefits. And with only 9% of Americans consuming the recommended five servings of fruit and vegetables per day, it is hard to think that optimal levels of vitamin C will be acquired through food alone.[112]

Unfortunately, most dietitians and physicians have only been made familiar with the benefits of vitamin C_1 and are unaware that vitamin C_2 even exists.

A new RDA for vitamin C for smokers has been established at 100 milligram per day, but this is like giving a soldier a baseball bat—better than nothing, but far from optimal. Even the most conservative estimates for smokers begin at 200 milligram per day, and smokers would benefit from doses far higher than that. Smokers who take optimal amounts of vitamin C and beta-carotene can reduce their risk for lung cancer. A better RDA for smokers would be 1,000 milligram per day.[113, 114, 115]

Vitamin C protects against virtually all forms of radiation. It powerfully prevents the damaging effects of X-radiation. It should be common practice for anyone undergoing X rays of any kind to supplement with vitamin C in the days and hours preceding their X rays.[116] Vitamin C has also been found helpful in reducing the damaging effects of ionizing radiation.[117] Anyone who spends significant amount of time in the sun needs to consume optimal amounts of vitamin C and other antioxidants for maximal protection against UV radiation.

Vitamin C has been extensively studied for its anticancer effects. It has more wide-ranging effects in preventing cancer than any other nutrient known.[118, 119] As long as there are optimal amounts of vitamin C in the body, damage to cell membranes that leads to cancer cannot occur.[120] Eighty-eight population studies demonstrated vitamin C's protective effect: The more vitamin C people consumed, the lower their risk for cancer was.[121]

Vitamin C regenerates two important antioxidants: vitamin E and glutathione.[122] Without vitamin C, many of the body's protective mechanisms break down. Vitamin C can be thought of as an overall first-line antioxidant and defense against cancer and all forms of free radical attack.[123]

Breast cancer is one of the most prevalent forms of cancer striking the female population. Research suggests that a significant number of these cancers could be prevented if women consumed more vitamin C.[124, 125, 126, 127, 128]

Two grams of vitamin C per day has been shown in double-blind studies to protect the bronchial airways and lungs from cold temperatures, hay fever, and smog from traffic fumes.[129]

Vitamin C in very high doses has been shown to be of significant benefit to AIDS patients. Twenty to 200 grams per day has been used by Robert Cathcart, M.D., one of the country's best-known vitamin C researchers. Improvements seen include higher T cell levels, an important indicator of immune function. Complications such as Kaposi's Sarcoma were improved and even eliminated in some cases when high doses of C were given intravenously.[130, 131]

Vitamin C is also a very important nutrient for diabetics. It is one of the most important nutrients for preventing the clogging of arteries that often occurs as a complication of this disease. It has been shown the more vitamin C diabetics ingest, the less damage high levels of sugar in their blood will cause.[132, 133, 134]

Dr. Frederick Klenner amassed extraordinary clinical experience using vitamin C in large doses orally, intravenously, and intramuscularly. He documented these benefits through many articles published in medical journals. Dr. Klenner's work shows conclusively that vitamin C should be part of every physician's frontline attack against a wide range of viral and bacterial infections. Dr. Klenner also believed through his years of practice that even before a diagnosis can be made, large doses of vitamin C should be used when a fever is present. Insidious viruses that otherwise might have proven fatal were often neutralized by the use of high-dose vitamin C. Dr. Klenner believed that sudden infant death syndrome could in fact be an aggressive virus that can, through its attack on respiratory control centers in the brain, lead to a swift and life-ending illness. He believed that all infants who present even the mildest symptoms of cold, flu, or viral infection should be given large doses of C by their physicians. He used high doses of vitamin C to cure viral hepatitis in as little as two days. He also used upward of 10 grams of vitamin C intravenously post-operatively with patients undergoing surgery, and achieved much quicker recovery times in his patients. He also found intravenous vitamin C to be an effective treatment for polio. Vitamin C in high enough doses completely neutralizes the free radicals caused by the polio toxin. It is these free radicals that cause the damage that leads to the debilitating effects of polio. If treated in the early, acute stage, very high doses of vitamin C can completely eliminate this condition. The sixty polio patients he treated all recovered completely. According to Dr. Klenner, "I have never seen a patient that vitamin C would not benefit."[135, 136, 137]

Two-time Nobel laureate Dr. Linus Pauling did more to popularize the use of vitamin C than anyone else. He believed that vitamin C deficiency is the main cause for heart disease and many other degenerative diseases that shorten our life expectancy. He believed that everyone should take five to ten grams per day of vitamin C. The medical community is beginning to catch up with him and practitioners like Dr. Frederick Klenner. Hopefully physicians will begin to use vitamin C more widely. It is one of the safest and most beneficial substances ever discovered.

Food sources for vitamin C include citrus fruits, strawberries, tomatoes, broccoli, peppers, leafy greens, and potatoes.

Vitamin C Guidelines

- Make sure to take a minimum of 500 milligrams per day of vitamin C. Optimal amounts range from 1 to 8 grams per day and beyond.
- Vitamin C should be taken throughout the day or in a time-released form to help your body tissues maintain optimal levels.[138, 139, 140]
- Buffered versions of vitamin C are fine for those who cannot tolerate the acidity of regular ascorbic acid. Dollar for dollar, however, there is nothing better than regular old ascorbic acid powder. Expensive "high-tech" vitamin Cs have no proven benefits over ascorbic acid.
- Vitamin C is extraordinarily safe and nontoxic.[141]

CHAPTER 15

Fat-Soluble Vitamins

BETA-CAROTENE AND VITAMIN A

Vitamin A comes in two forms: beta-carotene, found in a wide variety of fruits and vegetables, and vitamin A, found in liver, eggs, butter, cod liver oil, and fortified dairy products. Vitamin A adds color to the world. Beta-carotene gives plants, flowers, fish, and birds their many pigments. Vitamin A in our eyes allows us to see them.

For decades, researchers believed the only function of beta-carotene was to serve as a precursor to vitamin A. Yet recent research has shown that beta-carotene boosts the immune system, protects arteries from clogging, and prevents cancer. It is an important nutrient in its own right. Generous amounts of both nutrients are needed for optimal health.

Certain conditions, such as hypothyroidism, may limit the body's ability to transform beta-carotene into vitamin A. If you are a vegetarian or do not eat vitamin-A-rich foods and have low thyroid function, take a supplement with at least 5,000 international units of vitamin A per day. Since many have slightly low thyroid function, modest doses of vitamin A should be in almost every supplement regime.

Both vitamin A and beta-carotene are fat-soluble vitamins. They are stored and metabolized in the fatty tissues of the body. Only vitamin A poses even the remote possibility of toxicity, and only if taken in high doses over prolonged periods. Beta-carotene may turn skin orange if taken in high doses, but this is harmless. Alcoholics or those with liver damage, however, should avoid high doses of both forms of vitamin A. Impaired liver function does not allow us to metabolize these and many other nutrients correctly.

Vitamin A is needed for eyesight, healthy skin, the integrity of the intestinal tract, and for protection against pollution. Vitamin A's immune-boosting ability earned it the title "the infection vitamin" in the early part of the twentieth century. It's health-promoting ability was celebrated in a love song in the 1930s:

If I could hate ya
I'd run away
But that ain't my nature
I'm filled with vitamin A

("Young and Healthy," 1935)

Vitamin A is the most important nutrient for protection against cancers of the oral cavity.[142] A study showed that administering 32,000 IUs of vitamin A to tobacco chewers with oral leukoplakia for six months reduced the formation of new lesions and caused a complete remission of existing lesions in over 50% of the cases. Many studies have shown that specific nutrient deficiencies are just as strong a risk factor for developing cancer as destructive habits such as smoking and excessive alcohol consumption.[143]

Vitamin A has been found to be lower in children suffering from measles, a disease that kills two million children throughout the world each year. Every study examining children with measles finds low levels of vitamin A.[144] This has led researchers to consider low vitamin A levels a risk factor for measles. Studies have shown that putting children with measles on high doses of vitamin A for one week cuts the death rate in half.[145] Researchers suggest that children who have measles be given vitamin A whether or not they are deficient.[146, 147, 148]

Pregnant women or women who are trying to become pregnant should ingest no more than 8,000 IUs per day of vitamin A, either through supplements or vitamin-A-rich foods such as liver, milk, or cod liver oil. In large doses, vitamin A can cause malformations of the fetus. This does not mean that pregnant women should avoid vitamin A. Doses of 6,000 IUs have been used effectively in pregnant women who were deficient in this vitamin.[149] Pregnant women need vitamin A to make progesterone and other hormones. Beta-carotene may be the ideal form of vitamin A for pregnant women as it has no effects on the fetus.

Both forms of vitamin A are critically important for the smoker. Smoking lowers vitamin A levels in the respiratory tract even if there are adequate stores of vitamin A in the liver. Smokers need at least 25,000 IUs of vitamin A per day to compensate for this loss. Their need is far greater than that of nonsmokers.[150] Ideally, higher doses should be taken weekdays only. This gives the body two days off to metabolize the higher dose.[151, 152]

Research suggests that persons who suffer from gout should limit their intake of vitamin A. It may increase uric acid levels and worsen symptoms. Beta-carotene has no such effects and is the vitamin A of choice for gout sufferers.[153]

Short-term doses of vitamin A can range as high as 100,000 IUs for immune strengthening and fighting acute infections and viral diseases. Such doses are highly effective at fighting illness and encouraging wound healing but should not be carried out for more than two weeks. They should also not be taken without medical supervision or by a woman who has even the remotest chance of becoming pregnant. It should also be accompanied by at least 200 IUs of vitamin E. Vitamin E keeps vitamin A "fresh" in the body.

The best form for high-dose vitamin A therapy is the micellized version. Micellizing is a process of predigestion that allows fat-soluble vitamins to be absorbed without assistance from the liver. Since the liver is where vitamin A (not beta-carotene) can build up and cause problems when high doses are taken, bypassing the liver is a good idea.

Most unhealthy people have both suboptimal liver function and fat-digesting ability, which is why I recommend the micellized form more than any other.

Food sources for vitamin A include eggs, butter, liver, fish oils, and fortified milk, though I do not recommend fortified milk as it often gives the body too much vitamin D.

Vitamin A Guidelines
- If you are a smoker, chew tobacco, or breathe smog or other airborne pollutants, take a multivitamin with at least 25,000 IUs of vitamin A. For most people, 10,000 IUs of vitamin A should suffice.
- Those with low thyroid function do not convert beta-carotene into vitamin A well and require a regular intake of vitamin A through food or supplements.

- If you are pregnant or are trying to become pregnant, do not ingest more than 8,000 IUs of vitamin A per day.
- Higher doses of vitamin A should be accompanied by increased intake of vitamin E, which protects vitamin A from oxidation.
- Long-term high-dose vitamin A should not be taken without medical supervision.
- For therapeutic purposes, micel A is best.

Beta-Carotene

Beta-carotene is the star of the carotenoids, a family of over six hundred pigments that give orange and yellow produce their color. Even deep green vegetables like spinach and broccoli are loaded with carotenoids. The green chlorophyll content of these vegetables masks their yellow-orange carotenoids. When broccoli goes bad, it turns yellow. The chlorophyll oxidizes, revealing the yellow pigments underneath. Likewise, colorful fall foliage is filled with the many colors of carotenoids.

Beta-carotene was once only thought valuable due to its ability to be turned by the body into vitamin A. But beta-carotene has won respect in its own right as a powerful antioxidant, an important nutrient for a strong immune system, and for its ability to help maintain clear arteries and reduce the incidence of certain cancers.

Many studies have shown that beta-carotene levels are lower in tissues of cancer victims. The lower your beta-carotene levels, the greater your risk for cancer.[154] Beta-carotene protects against many forms of cancer, particularly cancers of the stomach, lung, colon, and breast.[155, 156, 157] Beta-carotene has also been shown to work with vitamin C in reducing the risk for cervical dysplasia and other premalignant lesions in the body.[158, 159, 160, 161, 162, 163]

If the palms of your hands turn yellow-orange when you drink a lot of carrot juice or take beta-carotene supplements, you have not developed beta-carotene toxicity. Yellow skin simply is a sign that you are storing it in the fat that is directly under your skin.[164]

Look for supplements that contain food-derived beta-carotene. If a supplement does not specify the kind of beta-carotene it contains, it is invariably synthetic. Synthetic beta-carotene is beneficial, but does not have the same molecular structure as the beta-carotene found in foods. It is often encapsulated with chemical preservatives. Natural food concentrates of beta-carotene do not contain such preservatives. And, like all food sources of beta-carotene, these natural preparations contain a variety of other carotenoids for more protective power. My favorite carotenoid supplements are those that feature the carotenoids of the sea plant Dunaliella salina or come from other natural food concentrates.[165]

Best food sources for beta-carotene include sweet potatoes, carrots, winter squash, broccoli, red bell peppers, tomatoes, dark leafy greens, apricots, mangos, and pink grapefruit. These foods are also loaded with vitamin C, bioflavonoids, and other protective antioxidant nutrients.

Beta-Carotene Guidelines

- Eat and juice as wide a variety of fruits and vegetables as possible. Steaming and lightly cooking vegetables allows us to absorb more beta-carotene from produce than eating it raw.
- Supplementing with at least 75,000 IUs is strongly recommended for those who avoid vegetables, breathe polluted air, have cataracts, smoke, live or work with a smoker, or who want to minimize their risk of cancer and heart disease.
- Supplements of beta-carotene should come from natural sources such as carrot concentrates and extracts of the sea plant *Dunaliella salina*. Optimal supplement intake ranges from 25,000 to 100,000 IUs per day, and should be balanced with other antioxidants.

Vitamin D

Many researchers would like to reclassify vitamin D as a hormone because of its powerful effects on the body. One of its most important jobs is to help calcium absorption. It also ensures that there is enough calcium in the blood for adequate bone formation.

Vitamin D has long been called the "sunshine vitamin." When your skin is hit with direct sunlight, it turns cholesterol into vitamin D. You can fulfill a year's requirement of vitamin D if you expose your face to twenty minutes of sunlight for only four months of the year. Sitting by a closed window does not help. Glass, clothing, and smog—but not clouds—block the ultraviolet rays that create vitamin D.

Those at risk for vitamin D deficiency include those who work at night, the housebound, those on ultra-low-fat diets, the elderly, and those on anticonvulsant medication. Strict vegetarians who never see the sun are also at risk. They may need vitamin D supplementation, or better still, regular, small amounts of sunshine.[166, 167, 168]

Low-fat diets for housebound elderly may place them at significant risk for vitamin D deficiency. Restricting fat can restrict intake of foods such as dairy products that contain vitamin D. This is not an ideal diet for seniors and others at risk of developing osteoporosis.[169]

Vitamin D deficiency is the most common nutritional deficiency in Crohn's disease. Between 30% and 68% of Crohn's patients have low levels of vitamin D.[170] If sunshine is not available many months of the year, supplementation may be needed.

Vitamin D in excess is harmful. Consumption of vitamin-D-fortified foods such as milk by those who regularly spend time in the sun is not recommended. Prolonged excessive doses of vitamin D calcifies tissues, accelerates aging, and causes heart disease and kidney damage.[171, 172] Those receiving high doses of vitamin D should do so only under the supervision of a physician who will monitor calcium and vitamin D levels.[173] Moderate, not excessive, sunshine is the best way to get vitamin D.[174] Research has shown that vitamin D derived from sunshine is superior to supplemental vitamin D in helping calcium absorption and promoting bone health.[175]

Vitamin D can be found in eggs, butter, fortified milk, and fish oil.

Vitamin D Guidelines
- If you spend twenty minutes per day in the sun during the summer, do not supplement with vitamin D or eat vitamin-D-fortified foods. If you have darker skin, you may require an hour of sun per day to meet your vitamin D requirements.
- If you are housebound or work at night and never see the sun, consume small amounts of fortified dairy products or cereals *or* take a multivitamin with 400 IUs of vitamin D.

Vitamin E

Vitamin E is another potent antioxidant nutrient that combats the effects of free radicals. You cannot get optimal amounts of this nutrient through food. Even those foods that used to contain small amounts of vitamin E—vegetable oils—have had their vitamin E removed. Refined vegetable oils actually deplete your body of vitamin E and increase your need to supplement. In order to get the wide-ranging protective effects of this nutrient, you need to supplement somewhere in the range of 100 to 800 IUs per day. Optimal intake of vitamin E has been shown to boost the immune system, reduce the risk of heart disease and cancer, prevent angina, and prevent the development of cataracts. Most Americans only get 12 IUs per day, far below the optimal range.[176]

Daily doses of vitamin E have been shown to reduce free radical damage and improve the action of insulin in diabetics.[177] Vitamin E has also been shown to protect the heart from damage that occurs when magnesium is deficient. Magnesium deficiency is widespread in America.[178]

Vitamin E is important for exercisers. It decreases the damage done to tissues that can occur from all forms of aerobic activity, including running, aerobics, or cross-country skiing. It is very important for older persons who are active, for they have a reduced ability to neutralize the free radicals created during exercise. Weight lifters also need to protect their tissues with vitamin E.

If you climb mountains or live high above sea level, you should also supplement with E. It protects the body from the damage that can occur at high altitudes when tissue levels of oxygen are low.[179, 180]

A Finnish study examined 36,000 adults during an eight-year period. During this time, 766 people in the group developed cancer. Those who entered the study with low levels of vitamin E had one and a half times greater risk of developing cancer compared to those with higher levels.[181] Vitamin E also decreases the risk of oral and pharyngeal cancer.[182] Vitamin E has been found to be low in women suffering from preeclampsia.[183, 184, 185] Researchers suggest that the amount of vitamin E found in most multivitamins, 30 IUs, is not enough to help prevent cancer, and recommend protective doses in the range of 100 to 400 IUs per day.[186]

Vitamin E protects the health and function of the nervous system more than any other essential nutrient.[187] Vitamin E may prevent the occurrence and slow the progression of Alzheimer's disease.[188, 189]

Vitamin E supplements are best taken with meals that have some fat in them unless one is taking a "micellized" or water soluble form. Micellized vitamin E supplements are far better absorbed and utilized than normal gel capsule versions, especially in those with serious illness or digestive disorders. This is not to say that capsules are not effective. They are beneficial and convenient. But for those who wish to have the maximum absorption and tissue saturation with vitamin E, micel E is best.

Unrefined vegetable oils, nuts and seeds have some vitamin E, but only enough to help manage their own unstable fatty acids. The only way to get optimal levels of this superstar nutrient is to supplement.

Vitamin E Guidelines

- Everyone should take vitamin E, especially those who smoke. Food does not supply enough. Optimal intake ranges from 400 to 800 IUs per day.
- Vitamin E may cause a slight increase in blood pressure in hypertensives. Those with high blood pressure should begin with no more than 100 IUs per day and should ideally take it under supervision of a health care practitioner.
- Vitamin E thins the blood, so anyone taking blood-thinning medication should only take vitamin E under medical supervision.
- While all forms of vitamin E are beneficial, natural vitamin E, d-alpha tocopherol, appears to have the most benefit.
- Those on ultra-low-fat diets or with fat absorption problems should use micellized vitamin E.

VITAMIN K

Vitamin K is a fat-soluble vitamin needed for blood clotting, bone formation, the regulation of blood calcium levels, and cancer prevention. Leafy greens are the only significant food source of vitamin K. The beneficial bacteria in the colon also manufacture it, fulfilling half of the daily requirement for this nutrient.

Antibiotics reduce the amount of vitamin-K-dependent clotting factors in the body. This occurs because antibiotics wipe out the beneficial bacteria that make vitamin K. Leafy greens should always be eaten during any period when antibiotics are prescribed. Long-term antibiotic use may dictate the need for supplementing with vitamin K.[190]

Vitamin K Guidelines

- Eat plenty of green leafy vegetables, particularly kale, parsley, broccoli, and turnip greens. Most vegetables have some vitamin K. Milk, soybeans, and eggs also contain some vitamin K.
- Supplement with vitamin K from 70 to 140 micrograms if you do not eat greens. This amount is found in most multivitamins.
- Talk to your doctor before supplementing with vitamin K if you take blood-thinning medication.

CHAPTER 16

Minerals

CALCIUM

Though most calcium is found in bone, calcium is also very important for many bodily functions. Calcium has been well documented for its ability to:

- Lower blood pressure in hypertensives[191, 192]
- Prevent colon cancer[193, 194]
- Nourish and calm the nervous system
- Enhance immune function by strengthening cell membranes

Calcium is one of the most important nutrients for the prevention of bone loss. This beneficial effect of calcium on bone health will only occur, however, when calcium is:

- Taken in amounts of 500–800 milligrams per day throughout life
- Balanced with all trace minerals and vitamins C, folic acid, and vitamin K
- Not antagonized by sugar, caffeinated coffee, smoking, or alcohol
- Not excreted due to consumption of more than 12 ounces of protein per day
- Not excreted due to consumption of sodas, diet and regular, which contain phosphoric acid
- Combined with adequate exercise, especially weight-bearing exercises such as walking, jogging, or aerobics

The current calcium supplementing program suggested for most women is incomplete. It is not balanced with other minerals and may be unhealthy. Supplementing with high doses of calcium alone impairs absorption of other trace minerals needed for bone formation such as zinc.

Dairy products are abundant in calcium. The phosphorus and specific proteins in dairy products, however, can take calcium from the body. This may explain why countries like the United States, Australia, and Scandinavian countries, which have the highest consumption of dairy products, also have the highest incidence of osteoporosis. Many are allergic or intolerant to dairy products, or may avoid them due to their high fat content.

Calcium Guidelines

- A total daily intake of at least 800 milligrams is recommended, balanced with other vitamins and minerals. Women need calcium in adequate amounts throughout their life, particularly between the ages of fourteen and thirty-five when they are laying down their lifetime stores of bone. More is needed during pregnancy, during times of stress, and to help heal bone fractures.
- Calcium carbonate is a fine, inexpensive source of calcium for healthy people with good digestion. Calcium citrate is better for those over age fifty who may not have sufficient stomach acid.
- Antacids are not recommended as a source of calcium. They contain toxic metals such as aluminum and can neutralize the stomach acid needed for calcium absorption.
- Avoid calcium supplements with vitamin D unless you are housebound or never go in the sun.
- Broccoli, cabbage, nuts and seeds, tofu, sea vegetables, green barley drinks, and leafy greens are also good sources.

MAGNESIUM

Magnesium is the number one mineral Americans are deficient in. According to the USDA, not only do most Americans not get the RDA for magnesium, most of us—56%—do not even get *two thirds* of that amount. Because magnesium is depleted by stress, exercise, and alcohol, our needs often go well beyond the RDA, which many find inadequate in the first place.[195]

Optimal levels of magnesium:
- Prevent kidney stones
- Lower blood pressure
- Build healthy bones

- Enhance athletic endurance and increase muscle size in response to weight training
- Protect the heart and arteries
- Relieve muscle cramps
- Protect the body from the damage of stress
- Increase energy production and fat burning
- Enhance insulin function
- Balance blood sugar
- Help relieve the nervous tension and low blood sugar of PMS
- Nourish and calm the nervous system
- Enhance immunity
- Prevent aluminum deposition in tissues
- Decrease cravings for foods such as chocolate

Magnesium is the most important nutrient for the heart. Getting optimal amounts of magnesium has been shown to:
- Increase cardiac output
- Prevent cardiac arrhythmias and deaths they cause
- Decrease the output of stress hormones, which in turn protects the heart[196, 197]
- Prevent the buildup of plaque on artery walls
- Prevent the dangerous depletion of magnesium caused by diuretic medications[198, 199, 200, 201, 202, 203, 204, 205, 206, 207]

Congestive heart failure patients frequently have low magnesium levels.[208] Most patients suffering from peripheral vascular disease are also deficient.[209] Magnesium is also excreted in higher amounts by those with mitral valve prolapse.[210, 211, 212, 213]

Magnesium deficiency is the most common mineral deficiency in diabetics. This causes many of the complications seen in this disease.[214] Magnesium and insulin work hand in hand transporting sugar in the body. Magnesium deficiency stops the body from using sugar correctly. Diabetics supplemented with magnesium have greatly improved sugar metabolism and tissue response to insulin.[215, 216] Type II diabetics have significantly reduced magnesium levels when compared to healthy controls. Low levels of magnesium may be one of the main reasons insulin fails to work for Type II diabetics.[217, 218]

Magnesium has been shown to be helpful in the treatment of viral and bacterial infections, bronchitis, acne, and conjunctivitis. It is also particularly important for those who suffer from an overgrowth of yeast known as candida albicans.[219, 220, 221, 222]

If you have enough magnesium in your blood, that does not mean you have adequate amounts in your body.[223] Serum magnesium is like the amount of money in your pocket. The amount in your tissues is like your net worth. The two have nothing to do with each other. Magnesium spends its time inside your cells, not outside. Serum levels of magnesium can be elevated and magnesium deficiency can still be present.[224] Red blood cell or white blood cell magnesium is a better indicator of body stores. The best test for magnesium, however, is the magnesium loading test. In this test, magnesium is administered orally or intravenously. A lack of magnesium in the urine is seen as a clear sign of deficiency.[225, 226, 227] This method has detected magnesium deficiency in a large percentage of hospital patients.[228]

Food sources for magnesium include nuts, seeds, whole grains, beans, seafood, leafy greens, and fresh vegetable juices. Few Americans eat enough of these foods.

Magnesium Guidelines

- Everyone should receive between 400 and 600 milligrams of magnesium per day through food or supplements. Those who exercise, are under stress, take diuretics, or are ill need more.
- Magnesium oxide, citrate, chloride, and aspartate are beneficial forms of this mineral.[229]
- Epsom salt baths are another way to get more of this valuable mineral into your body.
- Those with kidney failure or any serious medical condition should talk to their doctor before taking magnesium supplements.

POTASSIUM

The cells of the body are like rowboats in a stormy sea that are constantly pumping water overboard. Except what the cells of the body are trying to get rid of is sodium. They are trying to replace it with potassium. Keeping the right amount of these minerals in your cells is so important that your body expends more than one third of its energy trying to maintain this balance.

This is a balance that is increasingly harder to keep. Most Americans do not get enough potassium and eat too much sodium. Food refining and processing is to blame. The potassium naturally present in a large variety of natural foods is removed when whole grains are turned into white flour, apples are turned into apple juice, etc. They are then loaded with sodium compounds that give products shelf life and flavor. Since prehistoric times to the present, the ratio of potassium to sodium has been reversed. We need to eat ten times as much potassium as sodium. We now often eat more sodium than potassium. This imbalance leads to many problems:

- Bloating
- Fatigue
- Calcium excretion
- Arrhythmias
- Heart disease
- Cancer
- Hypertension[230]

It has been shown that food that is not organically grown is much lower in potassium than organically grown foods.[231] All the more reason to eat as many unrefined potassium-rich foods as possible, for our produce does not give us as much as it used to.[232]

Those on diuretic medications need to pay special attention to get as much potassium and magnesium in their diet as possible. These medications can lead to dangerously low levels of both of these nutrients.[233]

Potassium Guidelines

- While supplements of potassium can be helpful, the best way to get enough is to eat a diet of whole, unrefined foods, preferably organically grown.
- Nuts, fruits, potatoes, diary products, and vegetables are the best source for potassium.
- Potassium is found in virtually every food that has not been refined, including lean meats.
- Yogurt, ounce for ounce, has more potassium than a banana.
- Lightly steaming or juicing vegetables will help release more of the potassium they contain.

IRON

Roman soldiers added iron filings to their wine before going into battle to increase their energy and resilience. Iron is needed to make healthy red blood cells, which supply the body with oxygen. Without enough iron, immune function and energy levels decline. Yet iron requires careful attention to be of benefit. Too much and too little are equally undesirable.

Iron should not be taken at the same time as thyroid hormone. Iron binds thyroid hormone, rendering it ineffective. If you need both iron and thyroid hormone, which many women do, take them at different times of day. Those with low thyroid who are also frequently low in iron should consider taking vitamin A or increasing consumption of vitamin-A-rich foods. Low thyroid function can decrease the ability of the body to convert beta-carotene in fruits and vegetables into vitamin A. Vitamin A has a positive effect on iron metabolism, and has been shown to help increase iron blood levels.[234, 235, 236]

Menstruating and pregnant women often need additional iron. Children can be deficient, particularly those who suffer from learning disabilities. For men and postmenopausal women, however, iron supplementing or eating iron-fortified foods is not recommended. Because men do not experience blood loss and are mostly meat eaters, they rarely need iron supplements. Half of Americans have too much iron in their body. Over one million Americans have an inherited disorder that causes them to store too much iron. Excess iron causes considerable problems:

- Too much iron accelerates aging.
- Excessive body stores of iron increase the risk for heart disease.[237]
- Excess free iron creates free radicals, which cause cancer. Iron also feeds cancer cells directly.[238]
- Adults absorb less than 10% of ingested iron. The remainder takes days to travel through the colon if a low-fiber diet is consumed. This unabsorbed iron then reacts with fats in the undigested food and promotes colon cancer.[239, 240]
- In certain diseases, the body sequesters iron and creates anemia in order to keep iron away from viruses and bacteria. They require iron for growth. The well-meaning physician may then order iron supplementation or a transfusion. The condition will often worsen due to this increased iron load.
- The common practice of taking iron before surgery does more harm than good.

- Iron overload has been found in many persons with psychiatric illnesses and can cause or worsen their psychiatric problems. Excess iron will store in the central nervous system. A study of seven psychiatric patients demonstrated that when they were treated for iron overload, psychiatric behavior diminished significantly. In the months that followed the treatment, the symptoms did not return.[241]
- Researchers believe high levels of free iron in the brain may be one of the causes of Parkinson's disease.[242]
- Persons with infections of the gastrointestinal tract should avoid iron and iron-fortified foods during the course of their infection. Iron feeds pathogens that cause GI infections.
- Breast milk is far superior to iron-fortified formulas. Breast milk iron is protein-bound, and is better absorbed and much less available to microorganisms that cause GI infections.[243, 244]

Here are some important ways to keep iron beneficial:

- Consume adequate amounts of antioxidants such as vitamin C, E, beta-carotene, zinc, manganese, copper, and selenium that minimize free radical production from iron.
- Eat at least six ounces of protein per day. Protein keeps iron safely bound and beneficial.
- Avoid white flours, white rice, and enriched flour products. Consume only whole, unrefined grain products. These contain trace minerals and phytates that naturally limit iron absorption.
- Do not drink hydrogen peroxide. It encourages free iron to damage the GI tract.
- Avoid the use of cast-iron pots unless you are low in iron.
- Have serum ferritin tests performed annually.

The body has few exit routes for iron, and is very efficient at recycling it. Only blood loss, endurance exercise, and disease increase iron loss.[245, 246]

Iron has powerful effects on the body. It can create health, maximize oxygen concentration in tissues, and is necessary for optimal brain function. We have seen the problems associated with too much, but too little is just as undesirable. Too low a level of iron in the body can increase risk of certain cancers, such as cancer of the stomach.[247, 248] Iron is necessary for adequate energy levels, but don't take it merely be-cause you are tired. Too little and too much iron both cause fatigue.[249]

A serum ferritin test performed by your doctor is the only way to assess your iron needs. Until you know what you require, take an iron-free multivitamin and avoid all cereals and other foods fortified with iron. "Ferrous" is what iron is called on vitamin labels.

The best form of iron is heme iron found in animal products such as meat, chicken, and fish. These foods also have an unknown factor called MPF, which enhances iron absorption. Eating vitamin-C-rich foods or taking vitamin C supplements also enhances iron absorption. Heme iron from food cannot be absorbed in excess as easily as synthetic iron in fortified foods and supplements. Heme iron will also not increase the production of free radicals in the intestinal tract.[250] For the few who need it, the best iron supplement is a natural heme iron found in liquid liver extracts.[251, 252]

Food sources for iron include all animal products including meat, fish, poultry, and eggs, as well as legumes and dried fruits. The reason dried fruits have more iron than fresh fruit is that they are dried in iron containers.

Iron Guidelines

- Factors that increase iron absorption include vitamin C and other antioxidant nutrients, adequate stomach acid, and the MPF factor in meat, poultry, and fish. Heme iron from animal foods is the most absorbable form of iron.
- Factors that decrease iron absorption include coffee, tea, antacids, soy protein, manganese supplements, and fiber such as the phytates in whole wheat and wheat bran.
- Do not take iron without having a serum ferritin test performed by your doctor.
- Avoid all cereals and bread products fortified with iron, which includes all white "enriched" flour products.
- If you have a degenerative disease, such as diabetes, cancer, or heart disease, rule out high iron levels with a serum ferritin test.
- Keep all iron supplements and all multivitamins containing iron out of the reach of children.

ZINC

Zinc is one of the most important nutrients for immune function, blood sugar balance, and optimal health. Many zinc-rich foods, including red meat, nuts, and seeds, are avoided due to the erroneous belief that they are fattening or unhealthful. Zinc is quickly depleted by physical and emotional stress and alcohol consumption. Most Americans are deficient in zinc and need to supplement. Ninety percent of my clients do not have enough of this crucial mineral.

Zinc keeps our skin and our immune, nervous, digestive, and reproductive systems functioning optimally. Zinc is also a crucial nutrient for brain function. Zinc deficiency has been implicated in a range of neuropsychiatric disorders including epilepsy, multiple sclerosis, Huntington's disease, dyslexia, acute psychosis, schizophrenia, dementia, anorexia nervosa, attention deficit disorder, and depression. Zinc deficiency has also been implicated as a possible cause of Alzheimer's disease.[253]

All new tissue growth requires zinc. Zinc strengthens the membranes of our cells and helps them function optimally. This is very important for protection against a wide variety of diseases.

Zinc is also required for smell, taste perception, and adequate appetite. Food cravings, particularly for sugar and carbohydrates, can be caused or worsened by zinc deficiency.

The risk for cancer has been found to be significantly higher in those with low levels of zinc.[254] Zinc protects the liver from free radical damage, especially when taken as a supplement.[255]

Zinc is a crucial nutrient for diabetics. Diabetics have low levels of zinc and excrete it quickly.[256] Zinc prevents a wide range of diabetic complications by lowering and balancing blood sugar, helping insulin work more effectively, protecting insulin receptors on cells, helping the pancreas produce insulin, and by lowering cholesterol in diabetics as well.[257, 258]

Zinc is necessary for protein synthesis and for all wound healing. Zinc has been shown to cause an 83% improvement in the healing of leg ulcers when applied externally.[259] Zinc is a very important presurgery supplement.[260]

Macular degeneration effects 30% of Americans over age 75. It is the leading cause of vision loss among the elderly. Zinc deficiency may be one of the causes.[261] Doses of 100 milligrams per day have shown significant promise in helping delay the loss of vision associated with this disease. Such large doses should be monitored by a health professional and balanced with other trace minerals. High doses may be needed for older persons, as we do not absorb minerals as well when we age.[262, 263]

Long-term high doses of zinc are not recommended unless supervised by a health professional. Doses of zinc above 50 milligrams per day can lower copper levels, and copper is essential for normal cholesterol, blood sugar, and insulin metabolism. Always balance zinc supplements with copper in a 15-to-1 ratio.

Zinc is essential for all aspects of reproduction. Zinc is needed for ovulation and for the manufacture of sperm. Even mild zinc deficiency will lower men's testosterone levels. Perhaps oysters' high zinc content gave them their reputation as an aphrodisiac. In women, zinc deficiency can lead to spontaneous abortions, toxemia, growth retardation, and problems during delivery. Zinc has been found to be a very safe and beneficial supplement for pregnant women in doses of 10 to 60 milligrams per day.[264, 265]

Those suffering from anorexia nervosa have been found to have significantly lower zinc levels than healthy persons.[266] Zinc supplementation results in a significant increase in weight in those suffering from anorexia nervosa. Twenty females between the ages of fourteen and twenty-six who suffered from anorexia nervosa were given zinc supplements. Seventeen of them increased weight by more than 15%, and there was no further weight loss in any of the patients given zinc. Many studies show anorexia nervosa may be caused or worsened by zinc deficiency.

Low zinc levels may predispose one to chemical sensitivities. Fifty-four percent of those with such sensitivities to their environment are low in zinc. Zinc plays an important role in keeping toxic chemicals out of the body and protecting cells against the damage these toxins can create.[267]

Zinc is found in red meats, seafood, oysters, nuts, and seeds. The phytates in whole grains such as whole wheat may block zinc absorption.

Zinc Guidelines
- Tasting a solution of zinc sulfate heptahydrate is an excellent way to assess your zinc levels. Your taste reaction to this liquid will indicate whether you need zinc.

- Most who take zinc should take it in the range of 15-30 milligrams per day as zinc picolinate. Zinc gluconate is often ineffective.[268]
- When supplementing, balance zinc to copper in a 15:1 ratio.

COPPER

Optimal health requires just the right amount of copper. Both too little or too much of this double-edged mineral will cause degenerative disease. According to the USDA, Americans get only 50% to 60% of the recommended daily amounts.[269] Copper deficiency can cause:
- High blood cholesterol
- Increased blood pressure
- Elevated uric acid
- Increased blood insulin levels
- Unstable or elevated blood sugar
- EKG abnormalities
- Increased inflammation
- Anemia that will not respond to iron supplements
- Lowered immune function
- Increased risk of heart disease and osteoporosis[270, 271, 272]

Ceruloplasmin is an enzyme in the body made from copper. It is an important antioxidant and protects against a wide variety of free radicals.[273] Copper also stimulates higher levels of HDL cholesterol, the "protective" cholesterol, lowers LDL cholesterol, and helps the body maintain a favorable cholesterol ratio.[274]

Balance is crucial with copper. Copper in the right amounts participates in a powerful free-radical-scavenging enzyme known as superoxide dismutase. Excessive copper contributes to the production of free radicals. This is why there is no substitute for seeing a nutritionist who can assess your needs. Optimal copper levels are essential to controlling an overgrowth of candida albicans. A deficiency of copper has been found to limit the ability of white blood cells to kill candida,[275] while an excessive amount of copper will increase the pathogenic nature of candida albicans organisms.[276]

There are many factors that may explain why the French have a lower rate of heart disease than other developed nations. They eat less sugar and more fruits and vegetables than

Americans, and consume significant quantities of protective foods such as garlic and other antioxidant-rich herbs and spices. One of the other factors that may also protect them against heart disease is the liver, kidney, and other copper-rich foods they consume. Copper is also routinely sprayed on the grapes in French vineyards.[277]

Food sources for copper include meats, nuts (particularly almonds), and seeds.

Copper Guidelines

- Those taking zinc supplements for extended periods should take copper.
- In my experience, men often need copper, while women often have too much.
- Copper levels vary widely. One should ideally be tested before supplementing. Red blood cell copper can indicate low copper status. Only hair analysis can show excessive levels.
- The most beneficial, well-absorbed, and non-free-radical-producing form of copper is copper sebacate.[278, 279, 280]
- Supplement ranges for copper sebacate are from 1 to 3 milligrams per day, more if large doses of zinc are being consumed. Do not take copper at the same time as zinc or vitamin C.

MANGANESE

Manganese is an important trace element necessary for antioxidant defense, thyroid and brain function, and a healthy sugar metabolism. It is also needed for reproduction, bone and cartilage formation, and protection against osteoporosis. Dietary sources of manganese include nuts, seeds, whole grains, and organically grown leafy green vegetables. Even though only a few milligrams are needed each day, most Americans do not get enough. Our diet of meat, refined grain products, and chemically grown produce leaves us with a low intake of this essential mineral.[281]

Manganese is an important antioxidant nutrient. Manganese, like copper, is needed for the body to make a protective antioxidant enzyme known as superoxide dismutase (SOD).[282] Manganese also protects against the damaging effects of excessive iron.[283]

Manganese is a critical nutrient for sugar metabolism. Diabetics are usually deficient and benefit from supplementation.[284, 285, 286]

Manganese Guidelines

- Most benefit from 2 to 5 milligrams of manganese per day, the amount found in most high-quality multivitamins.
- Manganese can interfere with iron and calcium absorption.
- Long-term manganese supplementation must be balanced with other minerals.
- The best form of manganese is manganese picolinate.
- Long-term doses above 5 milligrams per day are not recommended without physician supervision.

CHROMIUM

Chromium helps the body use the hormone insulin more effectively. The benefits of optimal insulin metabolism are many. Chromium picolinate, the best absorbed and metabolized form of chromium, been shown to:

- Balance blood sugar and energy levels
- Eliminate sugar cravings
- Stimulate the growth of muscle tissue
- Lower body fat levels
- Lower triglycerides
- Lower total cholesterol
- Raise HDL cholesterol
- Lower LDL cholesterol
- Promote bone health

Studies have shown chromium can extend the life of rats. Finally, experiments even animal rights people can love: The animals lived 37% *longer* in the laboratory than they would in their natural habitat!

Chromium picolinate may extend life through its ability to slow a process called *glycation*—a damaging reaction in which sugar sticks like darts onto the proteins in our cells. Glycation is the process that makes the crust of bread, and is believed to be one of the factors that ages the body as well. (Is that where the expression "crusty old man" comes from?) By promoting lower sugar levels, chromium may extend life by reducing the amount of sugar that can participate in this damaging reaction.

Chromium picolinate may also slow aging through its ability to keep arteries clear and promote better circulation. When circulation declines to any part of the body, tissues are starved for oxygen and other nutrients. Free radical damage and cell death are then more likely to occur.[287]

Chromium enhances the ability of insulin to transport sugar into body cells.[288] It is not surprising, therefore, that chromium deficiency has been linked to diabetes and poor glucose tolerance. Chromium in adequate amounts may completely prevent adult-onset diabetes.[289, 290]

HDL is the most desirable cholesterol lipoprotein. It helps keep arteries clear. The ratio of HDL to total cholesterol is more important than the level of total cholesterol in predicting risk of heart disease. Chromium has been found to raise HDL 16% when 200 micrograms were taken three times per day.[291, 292, 293, 294]

Athletes have a higher requirement for dietary chromium. Exercise and an increased intake of carbohydrates both increase chromium losses. Chromium's ability to enhance the anabolic function of insulin helps it increase the muscle building effect of anabolic athletic training.[295]

Chromium Guidelines

- Everyone should take 200 to 600 micrograms of chromium per day.
- Brewer's yeast is the only food that supplies appreciable amounts of absorbable chromium.
- Chromium picolinate is well researched, nontoxic, and effective. It is the ideal form for supplementation.
- Insulin-dependent diabetics should take chromium under physician supervision, as it may decrease their insulin requirements.

SELENIUM

Selenium is another essential mineral needed in trace amounts for optimal health and disease prevention. When selenium goes into our body, it runs into a telephone booth Superman-style and emerges as glutathione peroxidase, quencher of free radicals, stopper of inflammation, booster of immune system, and remover of toxic substances. Glutathione peroxidase has also been found to decrease the incidence of heart disease, cancer, and multiple sclerosis. Not bad for something derived from a mineral needed in amounts of approximately 200 micrograms per day.

Most of us do not get enough selenium. Those eating low-protein diets may compromise their selenium intake even more.[296] Many researchers feel a great deal of disease is caused by low levels of selenium in our diet.[297, 298]

Studies from around the world have shown that where soil selenium levels are higher, there are significantly lower levels of cancers of the lung, rectum, bladder, esophagus, cervix, and uterus.[299] Studies from Finland have shown that male cancer patients have lower levels of selenium than healthy persons.[300] Breast and gastrointestinal cancer patients have also been found to be deficient. Selenium may be one of the most important protective nutrients against these forms of cancer.[301, 302]

Infants who suffered from sudden infant death syndrome have many signs of selenium deficiency. There is probably more to SIDS that selenium deficiency, but nursing mothers should take 100 micrograms of selenium per day to ensure adequate selenium for their children.[303, 304]

Selenium enhances mood levels in subjects given selenium supplements. It is not known whether selenium has a direct effect on the nervous system or improves mood by enhancing health generally. Differing amounts of selenium have been found in brain tissue, which suggests that selenium could act directly on the brain and nervous system.[305, 306]

Selenium has been found to be extraordinarily valuable in the management of acute pancreatitis. Supplementing with 500 micrograms per day of sodium selenite has saved the lives of those suffering with this ailment by stopping the progression of the disease. Improvement was seen as soon as twenty-four hours after supplements were taken.[307, 308]

Whole cereal grains, meat, and eggs are good sources of selenium. The amount of selenium in a food will depend on how much was in the soil it was grown in. Modern farming methods have decreased the amount of selenium available. Organically grown produce contains more than chemically grown foods.

Selenium Guidelines
- The recommended daily intake of 70 micrograms for men and 55 micrograms for women is not enough for

optimal health. Safe intake for selenium ranges from 100 to 400 micrograms per day.[309] Those consuming polyunsaturated vegetable oils such as sunflower, safflower, corn, and flax oil, and especially fish oils, have an increased need for selenium.[310]

- There are many beneficial forms of selenium. The best form for increasing the activity of the antioxidant enzyme glutathione peroxidase is sodium selenite. Vegetarians or those on low-protein diets may not derive much benefit from other kinds.[311, 312]

A Summary of Vitamin and Mineral Supplements

Supplement	Best form	Safe Intake Range
Beta-Carotene	Both synthetic and natural forms of beta-carotene have been shown to have protective properties. Natural preparations are better utilized by the body and may offer additional carotenoids for increased protective ability.	25,000–200,000 IUs per day.
Vitamin A	Vitamin A palmitate is fine, but micellized preparations absorb best and are recommended for acute conditions. Pregnant women or women who are trying to become pregnant should not consume more than 8,000 IUs of vitamin A per day. Excess vitamin A (but not beta-carotene) can have negative effects upon the fetus.	10,000–25,000 IUs per day is fine as a maintenance dose, with short-term medically supervised dosing up to 200,000 IUs possible.
B_1	Thiamine-HCL is fine, but the activated coenzyme preparation known as thiamine pyrophosphate may be more effectively utilized.	10–500 mg per day.
B_2	Riboflavin is fine, but some prefer riboflavin-5-phosphate, the coenzyme form.	10–100 mg per day.
Niacin	Regular niacin is fine for doses up to 250 mg per day. Higher doses should be in the form of no-flush niacin (inositol hexanicotinate), especially when niacin is being employed for cholesterol lowering. Other time-released forms are not recommended.	10–4,000 mg per day. Doses above 200 mg should ideally be done with medical supervision.
Niacinamide	Niacinamide	10–4,000 mg per day, with more than 500 mg per day requiring medical supervision.

Supplement	Best form	Safe Intake Range
Folic Acid	Folic acid	400–5,000 mcg. Pregnant women should take 800 mcg, but not more than 3,000 mcg. Take with B_{12}.
Pantothenic Acid	Pantothenic acid. When used as part of a total program to control blood lipids or to detoxify the liver, the activated form, pantethine, is recommended.	10–1000 mg per day.
B_6	Pyridoxine-HCL. P5P is an activated form that some may find more effective.	10–200 mg per day. Long-term doses above 200 mg per day require medical supervision.
B_{12}	Most people absorb B_{12} from animal products and probably do not need to supplement. For those who do supplement, hydroxycolbalamin is the superior form. For those who seek therapeutic effects from B_{12}, injections may be best.	50–5,000 mcg. Should always be taken with folic acid.
Vitamin C	Ascorbic acid works fine for most people. For those who cannot handle the acidity of ascorbic acid, use buffered versions such as calcium ascorbate.	500–8,000 mg and beyond, depending on individual needs and disease states.
Vitamin D	Should not be taken by those who receive 20 minutes of sunshine per day. The housebound should get 400 IUs from supplements or food per day.	Sunshine, or 400 IUs from food or supplements for the housebound.
Vitamin E	Alpha tocopherol is fine, but mixed tocopherols offer the most benefit. Micellized are best for optimal absorption and for acute conditions.	100–800 IUs per day. Those with high blood pressure should start with 100 IUs and do so under medical supervision.
Vitamin K	Best obtained in foods like leafy green vegetables.	Leafy greens, or 70 to 140 mcg per day.

Supplement	Best form	Safe Intake Range
Calcium	Calcium carbonate is fine for most people. Calcium citrate may be a better form for those over 50.	800–1,500 mg per day, depending on individual needs.
Magnesium	Most forms of magnesium work well. Citrate, aspartate, glycinate, and chloride are the best absorbed.	400–600 mg per day.
Potassium	Food is the best source, especially vegetables, vegetable juice, potatoes, or nuts.	99–500 mg per day when taken as a supplement.
Iron	Liquid Liver Extract and iron glycinate are two forms that work well without constipating. Anything that begins with the word "ferrous" is iron.	10–30 mg per day only for menstruating women or those with iron deficiency anemia. Pregnant and lactating women may need more.
Manganese	Manganese picolinate	2–5 mg per day. Doses of more than 5 mg per day require supervision.
Zinc	Zinc picolinate	15–150 mg per day. Doses above 75 mg per day should be supervised and balanced with copper.
Copper	Copper sebacate	Copper should be balanced with zinc in a zinc to copper ratio of 15:1.
Chromium	Chromium picolinate	200–600 mcg per day
Selenium	Sodium selenite	100–400 mcg per day

CHAPTER 17

Free Radicals and Antioxidants

I F HAULED BEFORE A JUDGE, free radicals would be accused of a wide variety of crimes. Heart disease, cancer, arthritis, Alzheimer's, Parkinson's disease, wrinkles, many varieties of cell death, and the process of aging itself all involve free radical damage. Free radicals do not pull off all of these jobs single-handedly, however. They have accomplices such as heavy metals, toxins in our food or environment, stress, overeating, and genetic tendencies. But free radicals do most of the damage.

In one way or another, free radicals are involved in the progression of almost every ailment. They are also one of the areas of our metabolism over which we can exert a significant amount of control. If we eat the right nutrients and adopt the right lifestyle, the body can limit their effects.

WHAT ARE FREE RADICALS?

Oxygen hates to be alone. When you burn food for energy, breathe smog, or have a stressful event in your life, you split a pair of stable oxygen molecules and create single bachelor oxygen radicals. These solo molecules then steal other molecules anywhere they can find them. This dating game continues until tissues are damaged. This can result in inflammation, cataracts, accelerated aging, depressed immune function, heart disease, or even cancer.

A Natural Byproduct of Your Metabolism
Free radicals cannot be completely eliminated by a healthy lifestyle. Some are formed by the natural everyday metabolism

of your body. Even those people who consume an optimal diet and have a healthy lifestyle create a certain amount of free radicals. They, too, have to ingest sufficient amounts of the protective nutrients that keep free radicals in check.

ANTIOXIDANTS: PROTECTORS OF THE BODY

Antioxidants neutralize free radicals. Without antioxidants, oxygen-based life-forms could not exist. The following nutrients have been found to have powerful antioxidant activity. Ranges of intake for maximum protection are suggested:

Nutrient	Preferred Form	Beneficial Ranges
Vitamin A	Micellized	10,000–25,000 IUs
Beta-Carotene	D. Salina or food-derived	25,000–200,000 IUs
Vitamin B$_2$	Riboflavin	10–100 mg
Vitamin C	Ascorbic acid or buffered versions	1,000–8,000 mg
Vitamin E	Mixed tocopherols	100–800 IUs
Magnesium	Magnesium oxide, chloride	400–600 mg
Zinc	Zinc picolinate	15–50 mg
Copper	Copper sebacate	1–2 mg
Manganese	Manganese picolinate	2–5 mg
Selenium	Sodium selenite	100–400 mcg
CoEnzyme Q10	– – –	25–100 mg
NAC	– – –	500–2,000 mg
Glutamine	– – –	500–3,000 mg
Taurine	– – –	500–3,000 mg

A chain is only as strong as its weakest link. For antioxidants to protect you effectively, they have to be balanced. An imbalance among them will significantly weaken your defense. For best results, work with a nutritionist who can test for your individual needs and make specific supplement recommendations.

Polyphenols and Bioflavonoids

Herbs, spices, fruits, and vegetables contain powerful health-modulating substances known as polyphenols and bioflavonoids. These substances have powerful antioxidant ability that is often many times more powerful than that of vitamins. They are one of the most exciting frontiers in preventive and therapeutic nutrition.

The following foods, herbs, and spices are rich in protective polyphenols and bioflavonoids:

- Cayenne or red pepper contains a powerful antioxidant known as capsiacin. Capsiacin is a very protective nutrient for the lungs. It is one of the most valuable substances for protecting against the damaging effects of cigarette smoke and smog.[313, 314]
- Thyme contains antioxidants and has long been used as a tea to help with coughs, bronchitis, and other immune problems.[315]
- Turmeric contains a powerful antioxidant that has been found to inhibit cancer in animal studies.[316]
- Rosemary contains potent antioxidants.
- Garlic quenches free radicals through its many sulfur compounds.
- Quercetin in apples and other foods has unique anti-inflammatory and immune-modulating effects.
- Milk thistle extract has glutathione-raising effects on the liver and protects the body from a wide range of toxins.
- The polyphenols in red wine are many times more powerful at preventing cholesterol oxidation than vitamin E.
- Unfermented green tea has powerful anticancer and liver-protecting properties.
- Proanthocyanidins found in grape-seed and pine-bark extracts are some of the most powerful antioxidants known.
- Other spices that have been found to have powerful antioxidant activity include cloves, cinnamon, cumin, fennel, and fenugreek.[317]

Antioxidants can only limit the amount of free radical damage that our cells undergo—they cannot stop it completely. Free radicals will always damage our bodies to some degree. The more antioxidant protection we have, the better. There is something that is even more important than getting a lot of antioxidants: preventing the formation of free radicals in the first place.

PREVENTING FREE RADICALS

It is exciting to see firemen extinguish blazing buildings and save lives through their heroism. Yet there is something even more exciting: eliminating the need for heroic rescues through fire prevention. The same is true for your body. Eating a lot of fruits and vegetables, consuming foods rich in bioflavonoids and polyphenols, and taking optimal amounts of vitamins C, E, and other nutrients should be a universal practice. But minimizing the radicals these nutrients need to quench is even more important. There are many things we can do to limit their formation.

Exercise

Cells will give off fewer free radicals when the body is regularly exercised. Exercise also puts more stable oxygen in your tissues. Poorly oxygenated tissues are actually more prone to the damage from free radicals than those with healthy amounts of oxygen.

Eliminate Toxic Metals

A hair analysis from a nutritionist or blood test from a physician will help show if you have toxic metals in your body such as cadmium, mercury, lead, and aluminum. High levels of iron and copper can also generate free radicals and should be checked for. These metals can all cause a significant amount of free radical damage. Avoid mercury dental fillings and do not use aluminum for food preparation or storage. Avoid aluminum-containing baking powders and antiperspirants, aluminum pots and pans, and antacids that contain aluminum. Switch to all-natural makeup that is free of aluminum and other toxic metals. Read labels.

Eliminate Toxins from Your Environment

Chlorine in water, pesticides on food, chemicals that come from office machinery, and the smog of urban environments all generate significant amounts of free radicals. Avoid all of them as much as possible.

Stress Management

Stress management is very important for reducing free radical formation. Overreacting, getting angry, and doing things in a frantic manner promote the formation of free radicals. Calm behavior is much less stressful on the body. This may be why type A personalities develop more diseases: They generate more free radicals through their behavior.

Maintain a Healthy GI Tract

A healthy colon produces far fewer free radicals. Consume bifidobacterium and acidophilus supplements as often as possible. Supplement your diet regularly with bifidobacterium-enhancing foods like FOS (see chapter 20). The colon is the site of the vast majority of free radical production in the body. Eliminating free radicals here will significantly reduce your body load of these destructive molecules.

Eat Yogurt

Fermented dairy products have many benefits. These foods promote health by helping populate the GI tract with the beneficial bacteria. They also contain modified fatty acids known as conjugated linoleic acid or CLA. CLAs stop the progression of free radicals the way a brick stops a line of falling dominos. By halting dangerous chain reactions, CLAs play a powerfully protective role. Even in low doses they offer significant protection. Indulge in sugar-free, plain yogurt with active cultures on a regular basis, with a small amount of fresh fruit added to liven it up. Never buy presweetened or artificially sweetened varieties.[318]

Eat Enough Protein

Protein is made of amino acids from which we make some of our most important antioxidants. Glutathione is a combination of three amino acids, and is one of the most powerful free-radical-neutralizing substances in our body. Glutathione not only scavenges free radicals but also helps eliminate a wide variety of damaging toxins that create them. NAC (N-Acetyl-Cysteine) is an amino acid supplement that helps the body make more glutathione.

Protein is needed to chaperone iron and copper throughout the body. When these essential minerals are bound to proteins, they are beneficial. But when there is a shortage of protein, as occurs during starvation or low-protein diets, these minerals can go into their free form and damage tissues.

Protein turns into protective enzymes in your body. CP-450 is not a World War II plane; it is the name of an enzyme your body uses to neutralize toxins. Undereat protein and you will not make enough. CP-450 has been found helpful in eliminating many toxic, free-radical-producing substances. Low levels of CP-450 have been associated with increased breast cancer rates. CP-450 is just one of the many guardian enzymes that are made from protein.

How much protein is enough? Two servings per day of at least 4 ounces of lean protein at lunch and dinner is sufficient for most people of about 150 pounds. A 4-ounce serving is the size of a deck of cards. Men and those under physical and emotional stress will need more; those with kidney failure, less. Eating your daily requirement of protein at one meal is not optimal. Divide your protein among as many meals as possible for maximum benefit.

Get Enough Sleep

Melatonin is a hormone released while you sleep. It is one of the most powerful scavengers of free radicals ever discovered. The reason sleep is so restorative is not only that it allows for tissue repair, but for free radical removal as well. Melatonin supplements are available but are not recommended for long-term use. Adequate rest and a healthy diet will give you enough melatonin.

Drink Plenty of Water

Water is needed in adequate amounts to absorb the damaging effects of an excited form of oxygen called singlet oxygen. Without adequate water, the energy of singlet oxygen cannot be absorbed as heat and will increase tissue damage from free radicals. The elderly and athletes often do not drink enough. Drink water regularly whether you are thirsty or not.

Don't Get Too Much Vitamin D

Vitamin D is important for healthy bones and teeth. That is why we have fortified dairy products with it. Yet too much vitamin D can lead to tissue calcification, which results in organ and artery damage. If you receive twenty minutes of sunshine per day, you are easily getting enough of this vitamin. Most people should avoid vitamin D supplements and fortified foods. Only if you are housebound and never see the sun should you consume vitamin-D-fortified foods or supplements.

The Good Side of Free Radicals

Free radicals are not always bad. Their powerful ability can be focused like prisoners on a chain gang to perform many tasks in the body. The cells of the immune system use tightly focused beams of free radicals to destroy invading viruses and bacteria.

Pregnant women release free radicals to stimulate the cells of the fetus to differentiate and turn into different organs. Athletes depend on free radicals to help them increase the strength of their muscles. Muscles damaged by free radicals created during exercise are stimulated to grow back stronger.

Longevity Nutrients?

Antioxidants will not assure you of 120 years. Antioxidants lengthen life as do safety belts: They prevent needless damage that leads to an early death and lower quality of life. Antioxidants from food and supplements should be taken in optimal, balanced amounts. The strength of their balanced protection will do a great deal to ward off premature death from unnecessary degenerative diseases such as heart disease, cancer, and other diseases caused or accelerated by the presence of free radicals.

CHAPTER 18

The Health Benefits of Garlic

G ARLIC IS THE MOST STUDIED herb in history. It has more benefits than any other single food. Tradition has told us that garlic has beneficial effects on health and longevity, and science is beginning to validate many of these claims.[319, 320, 321, 322]

At the First World Congress on the Health Significance of Garlic and Garlic Constituents held in Washington in August of 1990, over fifty scientists from around the world gave presentations demonstrating garlic's ability to prevent heart disease, fungal overgrowths, and infectious diseases. Other benefits of garlic discussed at this symposium included garlic's ability to remove toxic metals from the body and garlic's powerful antioxidant and anticancer effects. Over two hundred compounds are found in garlic, many of which are beneficial.[323, 324]

Studies of populations show that those who frequently consume garlic and onions have a lower incidence of cancer, which may be due to any number of the hundreds of sulfur compounds and trace minerals found in garlic.[325]

Garlic has also been found to have antibiotic and antifungal activities. Aged garlic extract enhanced the elimination of candida albicans in an animal study. Aged garlic extract has also been shown to prevent the powerfully carcinogenic mold aflatoxin that often contaminates peanut crops from attaching to DNA and causing cellular damage in humans.[326]

Differing methods of preparation will alter the way garlic effects the body. Many people claim allicin is the active ingredient in garlic. Allicin is a very short-lived compound that is

137

formed when garlic is crushed and soon changes into other substances. There are many beneficial substances in garlic, and attention should not be paid to allicin alone. Many of the supplements that claim to have significant amounts of allicin often have none.

Garlic's many sulfur compounds are the source of much of the immune-enhancing, detoxifying, and antibiotic properties of this amazing plant. These sulfur compounds are also powerful antioxidants that protect against the damaging effects of free radicals. It is this inhibition of free radicals that is part of the reason garlic is such a powerful protector against heart disease, cancer, and other ailments.

LOWERING BLOOD PRESSURE

Garlic is one of the most effective natural agents for lowering blood pressure. When blood pressure is too high, it can increase our risk for heart disease and stroke, and can damage many organs and tissues. Garlic has been found to lower both diastolic and systolic blood pressure when consumed regularly.

BOOSTING THE IMMUNE SYSTEM

Garlic has been found to be an important stimulator of the body's defense system known as the immune system. Garlic's sulfur compounds enhance the function of our defender cells known as white blood cells. White blood cells function more effectively when the body is supplied with antioxidant nutrients like garlic's sulfur compounds. Other immune-boosting elements in garlic include selenium and other trace minerals. Garlic also has direct antiviral and antibacterial properties. It also removes toxic heavy metals such as mercury that impair immune function.

BALANCING BLOOD SUGAR

Garlic has been shown in many studies to lower blood sugar in those who have high blood sugar levels. This is very important for diabetics, who often take medication to keep blood sugar under control. Hypoglycemics or those with low blood sugar should avoid large amounts of raw garlic, as it may lower their blood sugar even further and lead to fatigue. Aged garlic extract, however, has not been shown to have this effect, and is the garlic of choice for those with hypoglycemia.

PREVENTING HEART DISEASE

Garlic is one of the most important foods we can consume to lower our risk of heart disease. At the Fourth International Congress on Phytotherapy in Munich, Germany, in 1992, Dr. Jorg Grunwald concluded that garlic protects the heart and arteries in two ways:

1. Garlic reduces the free radicals that cause damage to cholesterol. If LDL cholesterol is not damaged, then it is harmless. When free radicals damage LDL cholesterol, it goes out of control and damages artery walls. The initial scarring that results and the presence of altered cholesterol molecules trigger the immune system to attack the damaged site on the artery wall, further enlarging the blockage. If LDL isn't oxidized, this process can be inhibited.

2. Garlic also inhibits the infiltration of damaged fats and cholesterol through the walls of our arteries. If cholesterol is so overabundant at one site that it tries to push its way through an artery wall, or a damaged LDL cholesterol molecule tries to damage an artery, garlic can inhibit this process.

This two-leveled protection is impressive. Add to it garlic's ability to lower cholesterol, triglycerides, and blood pressure, and garlic's ability to keep platelets from forming dangerous clots, and we can see why garlic is the single most important food for protecting the heart and arteries. Garlic is so effective at heart and artery protection that in Germany deodorized garlic supplements are licensed as drugs against atherosclerosis.[327, 328]

INTERMITTENT CLAUDICATION

Studies have shown that garlic is very effective at improving circulation in areas of the body where blood flow may be impeded due to clogged arteries. Thirty-two patients were studied over a twelve-week period. Those who supplemented their diet with garlic were able to significantly increase their walking distance after five weeks. Their blood pressure, cholesterol, and levels of spontaneous clots also decreased significantly.[329]

CANCER PREVENTION

In China and Italy and cultures where garlic is consumed, cancer rates are lower. Many laboratory experiments have shown that garlic is a powerful inhibitor of cancer. Both fresh garlic and aged garlic extract have been shown to have this effect.[330]

AIDS

Garlic has been found helpful in increasing the levels of immune cells in AIDS patients. After six weeks of treatment with aged garlic extract, the majority of the group studied saw the activity of their natural killer cells increase from dangerously low to normal levels. Symptoms such as diarrhea, candidiasis, and genital herpes all showed clinical improvement.[331]

WHICH FORM OF GARLIC IS BEST?

For regular consumption, it has been found that it is more beneficial to take a deodorized, aged garlic extract. There are many benefits to aging garlic:

- Deodorizing garlic removes its unsociable odor.
- The harsh, irritating properties of garlic are removed so that gastric irritation will not result.
- The valuable sulfur compounds found in garlic are more easily assimilated.
- Aging garlic enhances its antioxidant and immune-boosting properties.

Raw garlic may be too irritating for the GI tract of some people, and it also may cause sharp dives in blood sugar in hypoglycemics. For this reason, not to mention the odor of raw garlic, I recommend aged garlic extract for everyday use.

A SUMMARY OF GARLIC'S MANY BENEFITS:

- Garlic has been shown to have powerful immune-boosting properties and may be valuable in fighting off viral infections such as the common cold.
- Garlic has been shown to help lower blood pressure in those with hypertension.
- Garlic works as a natural antibiotic and reduces the number of harmful bacteria in the body.

- Garlic reduces blood cholesterol and triglyceride levels, and has been shown to limit the deposition of plaque on artery walls.
- Garlic has been shown to help the body eliminate parasites.
- Garlic reduces the amount of the yeast candida albicans in the human GI tract and has been shown to be beneficial in fighting systemic yeast infections.
- Aged garlic extract has been shown to promote the growth of beneficial bacteria.
- Garlic has been shown to lower blood sugar and be of significant benefit to diabetics.
- Garlic has been shown in population and laboratory studies to help prevent a wide variety of cancers.
- Garlic contains selenium, a cancer-preventing, immune-boosting, and anti-inflammatory nutrient.

CHAPTER 19

Top Ten Supplements

EVERYONE HAS A DIFFERENT METABOLISM, so it is difficult to say which supplements would be most important for you. For many people zinc is important, but it must be balanced with copper to suit your individual needs. Beta-carotene is a very important antioxidant, but if you eat five servings of fruits and vegetables per day, you would be better off spending money on a different nutrient.

Many of the antioxidant nutrients are available in one capsule. This is an especially good idea since it is better to have enough of all antioxidant nutrients than a lot of just one or two. This is convenient and may be best for most people.

If you are diabetic, have a heart condition, kidney problems, or are on blood-thinning medication, it is best to consult with your physician before starting a supplement program.

1. **Beneficial bacteria** such as acidophilus, bifidobacterium, and bulgaricus are the single most important supplement for overall health. If you do not have the right bacteria in your GI tract, you will not absorb vitamins, minerals, and other nutrients listed below or in your food optimally. Beneficial bacteria also greatly diminish free radical formation in the GI tract. More free radicals are produced in the GI tract than anywhere else in the body. Beneficial bacteria are important for immune function, protection against disease-causing bacteria, and for protection against food poisoning. Use high-quality refrigerated products.

2. **Vitamin C** is the most important antioxidant nutrient for the human body. Take at least 500 milligrams per day. A time-released 1,000-milligram supplement at breakfast and dinner would be best for most people.

3. **Vitamin E** is the fat-soluble antioxidant that everyone needs. Start with 100 IUs and build up to 400 to 800 per day. D-alpha tocopherol or mixed tocopherols are best. Take with a meal that has some fat in it.

4. **Magnesium** is a mineral that very few get enough of. Take 400-600 milligrams per day with meals. Add a cup of Epsom salts (magnesium sulfate) to your bath.

5. **Chromium** picolinate, 200–600 micrograms per day.

6. **Ginkgo biloba** standardized extract is recommended for everyone who can afford it. This herbal extract is one of the most important foods for optimizing circulation throughout the body and for maximizing brain health. Take 40 milligrams one to four times per day before meals.

7. **Milk thistle** standardized extract enhances liver function and is a powerful antioxidant as well. Take 100–200 milligrams per day before meals.

8. **NAC** (N-Acetyl Cysteine) is one of the most powerful antioxidant nutrients known. Start with one 500-milligram capsule on an empty stomach, and increase to two per day. Not recommended for diabetics without medical supervision.

9. **Niacin** in small doses is recommended for everyone as an antisenility nutrient. Take 50–100 milligrams per day with a meal. Harmless flushing of the skin may occur above doses of 50 milligrams.

10. **CoEnzyme Q10** is one of the most important all-around nutrients for heart health. It is important for healthy arteries, a strong heart, optimal immune function, and abundant energy, and can also help weight loss. Between 30 and 100 milligrams per day in the morning before breakfast is beneficial for most people.

Part III

Body Health

CHAPTER 20

Optimal Digestion for Optimal Health

You are what you absorb.

—Jeffrey Bland, Ph.D.

Y OU CAN TAKE SUPPLEMENTS, EXERCISE, eat well, and get adequate rest, but without optimal digestion, you cannot be healthy. The digestive system is not a mailbox where the food dropped in automatically reaches its destination. It has to be well nourished and free of the assaults of an unhealthy diet. It must produce a series of well-coordinated secretions. And it requires the right bacteria. Only then will it be able to absorb the nutrients you need to achieve optimal health.

It is easy to weaken the digestive system. If you have been assaulting your GI tract with overeating, inadequate chewing of food, alcohol, coffee, smoking, sugar, white flour, a lack of fiber, antibiotics, or eating under stress, you may have already significantly weakened your digestive ability. Many people feel they have a "cast-iron stomach" and eat as they please. The stomach is more like a velvet pouch. It and the rest of the GI tract do not respond well to repeated insults.

Many ailments can be caused or worsened by poor digestive function:

- Diverticulitis
- Varicose veins
- Osteoporosis
- Poor immune function
- Asthma
- Ulcers
- Heart disease
- Lowered immunity
- Macular degeneration

- Food allergies
- Candida overgrowth

Focusing on the GI tract to maximize health is not new. In the nineteenth century, naturopathic physicians gave the digestive function their full attention. The phrase "death begins in the colon" comes from their focus on this area of the body. Current-day physicians and nutritionists are beginning to once again understand that optimal health begins in the digestive tract.

Food goes through many steps before you digest and absorb it:

- You chew it adequately.
- Your digestive system secretes the right substances in the right amounts (stomach acid, buffers and enzymes from your pancreas, and bile from your liver/gallbladder).
- The wall of your small intestine facilitates the absorption of nutrients while keeping out pathogens.
- The liver and gastrointestinal lining transfer and metabolize nutrients so you can use them.

Chew

If you do not break down food into small enough pieces by chewing, food does not have enough surface area exposed to the digestive juices for digestion to occur. A block of ice will take all day to melt if you leave it in the sun. The same amount of crushed ice will melt quickly. Chewing food thoroughly—well past the point of sensory enjoyment—is essential if you are to get the most out of the food you eat.

Hydrochloric Acid

When food arrives in the stomach, it is met by hydrochloric acid and pepsin. These two secretions begin to break down the structure of the food so that the pancreas can finish the job. Good stomach acidity is essential to protein and mineral digestion. Unfortunately, many people, including half of those over age sixty, do not make enough stomach acid.

Insufficient stomach acid allows pathogens to enter your system that otherwise would have been killed. It also predisposes you to an ulcer. Ulcers are now thought to be largely due to the bacterium helicobacter pylori. When there is a shortage of stomach acid, this bacterium survives the passage through the stomach and can create an ulcer.

Hydrochloric acid insufficiency can be confirmed by a test from your physician. Do not take hydrochloric acid (HCL) unless you are sure you need it. Never take it on an empty stomach or if you have an ulcer.

Baking Soda

Baking soda is made not only by Arm & Hammer but by your pancreas as well. When food leaves the stomach and enters the small intestine, the body needs to not only neutralize the strong stomach acid, it needs to turn the food into the opposite of an acid state, called alkaline. Baking soda, which scientists call sodium bicarbonate, is an excellent buffering agent. Sodium bicarbonate is secreted by the pancreas onto the food that enters the small intestine. Only in an alkaline environment do pancreatic enzymes break down food. For this reason, sodium and potassium bicarbonate have been used as a folk remedy to enhance digestion. While there may be benefit from taking small amounts of such buffers one to two hours after a meal in a glass of water, it should only be done with the guidance of a health professional.

Constipation

Constipation is easily solved by avoiding refined white flours and increasing whole grain, vegetable, fruit, nut, and seed consumption. Do not use laxatives on a regular basis. They weaken bowel function and create a dependency. Increasing fiber in the diet, drinking more water, consuming flax oil, increasing magnesium intake, exercising, and checking for low thyroid function are the best ways to solve and prevent this problem.

Fiber

Americans eat only one third of the fiber they need. A lack of fiber has been implicated in causing many diseases of the gastrointestinal tract, including appendicitis, hiatal hernia, hemorrhoids, diverticulosis, varicose veins, colorectal cancer, diabetes, and heart disease. Increasing your intake of fiber is one of the simplest and most important things you can do to improve your health.

Fiber is the portion of plant food that is not absorbed and used for energy. Don't think this means that fiber serves no purpose. Fiber keeps our intestinal tract clean and functioning correctly. Fiber, especially insoluble fiber, is metabolized by intestinal bacteria into substances that prevent colon cancer. Fiber also dilutes and speeds the removal of toxins in food so that they minimally affect the delicate lining of the GI tract. Fiber is found in whole grains, beans and legumes, fruits, vegetables, nuts and seeds. Meat, fish, eggs, cheese, and all dairy products are devoid of fiber.

Two Families of Fiber

The kind of fiber that can dissolve in water is called soluble fiber, short for water-soluble. Foods high in this water-dissolvable fiber include oats and oats bran, barley, psyllium husks, flaxmeal, beans, peas, and many fruits and vegetables, such as carrots, citrus fruits, and apples. This kind of fiber has been associated with lower cholesterol levels and may help control or even prevent diabetes. Fiber that does not dissolve well in water—insoluble fiber—is found in such foods as wheat bran, corn bran, celery, and the skins of fruits and root vegetables. Insoluble fiber reduces the risk of intestinal cancers and helps prevent constipation and diverticulitis. Most whole foods contain a variety of fibers.

Which Kind of Fiber Is Best?

The best kind of fiber is whatever form is most convenient for you to eat. If you can include at least three to six servings per day of high-fiber fruits, grains, and legumes, you will receive all the fiber you need. Flaxmeal is the best food supplement for fiber. Organic flaxmeal is far superior to psyllium husk powder. The psyllium plant is sprayed with many undesirable pesticides.

Increase your intake of fiber-rich foods slowly, and combine it with an increase in water consumption. Six 8-ounce glasses of water per day is the absolute minimum needed for a smooth-running digestive tract.

Bitters

Bitter herbs have been used for centuries as a digestive tonic. Bitter foods tonify the liver and other digestive organs and help them produce more of the juices that help us break down foods. Salads eaten before meals were originally bitter greens that stimulated digestion. Coffee, unsweetened chocolate, and the occasional bitter greens are the only bitter foods left in the American diet.

Bitter foods do not make your digestive system lazy or lower their function as the long-term use of digestive enzymes can. Bitters enhance the function of the digestive glands by nourishing and tonifying them. Their effects are cumulative and positive. Examples of digestive tonic herbs include ginger, gentian root, and orange peel. Ginger has been found to have a powerful digestive enzyme known as zingibain.[332]

Should You Drink Liquids with Meals?
Studies have shown that in healthy persons, small amounts of liquids with meals enhance digestion by encouraging the secretion of more digestive juices. Healthy digestive glands hold a sevenfold reserve of their secretions.

Avoid Stress Eating
Never eat under stressful conditions. A relaxed eating atmosphere is essential for adequate blood flow to the GI tract. Eating while driving, arguing, or engaged in any other activity pulls circulation away from the abdominal region. Shifting blood flow in and out of the digestive tract is damaging. It creates free radicals that can decrease digestive function. Over time, this can lead to digestive inefficiency and thinning of the gut wall.

The Right Bacteria
Your intestinal tract is a zoo and you are the zookeeper. You have one hundred trillion bacteria in your GI tract, more than the number of cells in your body. The kind of bacteria you house plays a large part in determining how healthy you are. Friendly bacteria keep the immune system strong and the digestive system functioning smoothly. The wrong bacteria set the stage for disease. Friendly bacteria are always in the minority in the GI tract, but enough of them will keep the less beneficial forms that are always present from causing problems.

Beneficial bacteria:
- Help the body absorb all of the nutrients in food and supplements
- Help eliminate overgrowth of candida albicans
- Decrease cancer risk
- Lower cholesterol levels
- Boost the immune system
- Eliminate constipation, gas, and bloating

- Relieve skin problems
- Create vitamins
- Prevent/limit the severity of food poisoning, salmonella, and traveler's diarrhea[333, 334]

Think of your GI tract as a large city. You have two types of people in a city: the people who live there, and the tourists who pass through every day. Both are essential for the life of a city, and both the right residential and "tourist" bacteria are needed for the health of the GI tract.

Acidophilus and bifidobacterium are the two predominant residential beneficial bacteria in our intestinal tract. Both are essential to GI tract health. Yogurt and other fermented dairy products may or may not have acidophilus, depending on which brand you choose. "Active yogurt cultures" could refer to any number of bacteria, and does not necessarily mean acidophilus is present.

Although acidophilus is the bacteria most people are familiar with, bifidobacterium appears to be the most important beneficial bacteria in the GI tract. Bifidobacterium—which some may refer to by the outdated name "bifidus"—are particularly important for helping eliminate the overgrowth of candida albicans in the GI tract.

Bulgaricus is a beneficial tourist or "transient" form of friendly bacteria. It takes up to fourteen days to see all the sights in your GI tract. During its two-week voyage, it helps boost the health of your digestive system in many ways. It eliminates unfriendly bacteria, may prevent cancer, and has even been found to have antiherpes virus activity. It can be found in certain yogurts and high-quality supplements.[335]

There are at over two hundred strains of acidophilus, many kinds of bifidobacterium, and only certain strains of each have been shown to be of benefit. The consumer has no way of knowing when buying yogurt, acidophilus, or bifidobacterium supplements whether (1) the strains present are the ones that have been found beneficial in research or (2) whether the supplements even contain beneficial bacteria at all. Your best bet is to stick with high-quality manufacturers that sell their products in powdered, refrigerated form. Don't buy the cheapest probiotics, because you are likely to get what you pay for. The powdered, refrigerated versions are especially important for supplements of bifidobacterium and bulgaricus. Keep your probiotics refrigerated but never frozen.

Avoid chlorinated water; the chlorine will kill off beneficial bacterial in your GI tract. For GI health, drink only filtered, spring, or distilled water.

FOS

Fructooligosacharrides (FOS) are a complex of sugars that the body cannot digest. They are found naturally in foods such as bananas, onions, and Jerusalem artichoke flour, and are available as a supplement in powder or syrup form. They are an excellent food for bifidobacterium, which break them down and use them for growth. The sugars and starches we eat feed all the bacteria in your GI tract, good or bad. FOS are a targeted food that preferentially nourish certain strains of bifidobacterium without helping yeastlike organisms like candida. FOS taste mildly sweet, and may be the ideal replacement for sugar. For long-term maintenance of healthy bacteria in your system, a little FOS goes a long way. One quarter teaspoon consumed daily for four weeks has been shown to increase bifidobacterium population fivefold.

Antibiotics

Antibiotics upset the population of the bacteria in the GI tract. They also thin the wall of the GI tract, which can result in decreased integrity and function of the small intestine. Always combine antibiotic therapy with:

- Acidophilus and bifidobacterium taken at different times of day than the antibiotics
- Fibers that nourish the bowel wall such as apple pectin
- A sugar-free diet rich in leafy green vegetables

NUTRIENTS FOR THE HEALTH OF THE GI TRACT

A wide selection of vitamins and minerals is needed for a healthy GI tract. Many of the cells of the digestive tract live only seven days. They need many nutrients to reproduce quickly and without an error in cell reproduction that can lead to cancer. A high-potency, iron-free multivitamin as well as extra amounts of vitamins A, C, E, folic acid, and pantothenic acid will help keep the GI tract optimally nourished.

Zinc

Zinc is extremely important for the health of the entire gastrointestinal system. It is needed by ulcer sufferers, especially those on Xantac. Xantac reduces stomach acid levels, which in turn limits zinc absorption.[336] Without zinc, ulcers cannot heal. Xantac and similar medications may be effective for short-term management of excessive acid production, but in the long run delay the healing process.

Glutamine

Glutamine is an amino acid that is one of the most important nutrients for healing the GI tract. It has been found to be very helpful for ulcers, diarrhea, inflammatory bowel disorders, and all forms of intestinal repair. Typical doses range between 1 and 2 grams per day on an empty stomach.[337]

A Word for Travelers

If you are going to Mexico or any country where the water is of questionable quality, enhancing the health of your GI tract before leaving is of the utmost importance. Unfriendly bacteria and parasites have a more difficult time creating problems if you have beneficial bacteria in your GI tract. Three weeks before your trip, start supplementing daily with bifidobacterium. When on vacation, avoid the water. But if you do come in contact with a pathogen, you will have a much lower chance of feeling its negative effects if you optimize the health of your GI system beforehand.

CHAPTER 21

Boosting Your Energy Naturally

T HE BODY STARTS LIFE WITH abundant energy. Overwork, poor nutrition, glandular decline, and a buildup of toxins slow the body down. Most people's solution? Use stimulants. Coffee, sugar, cigarettes, and over-the-counter or illicit drugs are the most popular. These only worsen the problem. Consistently high energy levels can only be achieved by removing toxins from the body while increasing intake of nutrients to optimal levels. Real energy is the byproduct of optimal health.

Our goal in the pursuit of higher energy levels is to understand where the body's energy comes from, and get more energy by building up the body, not by destroying it further. Fatigue is a symptom of many ailments. If your energy declines suddenly, see your doctor and do not try to treat yourself. Rule out low thyroid function, iron overload, and other medical problems first.

Optimal levels of energy are only possible when the body is allowed adequate rest, not polluted with toxic foods and chemicals, and is given all the nutrients it needs to turn food into energy. Your quest for more energy should begin not by asking what will speed you up. You should look first for what is slowing you down. Many things get in the way of energy production:

- Impaired thyroid function
- A buildup of toxins throughout the body
- Vitamin, mineral, and essential fatty acid deficiencies
- Suboptimal liver function
- An overgrowth of yeast in the GI tract

155

- A lack of deep sleep
- Parasites
- Inadequate exercise
- Food allergy or intolerance
- Many illnesses and disorders

TOXINS IN THE BODY: THE MAIN CAUSE OF FATIGUE

City dwellers hate a garbage strike. Trash builds up on the corner and the whole neighborhood develops an unpleasant smell. The same thing happens when toxins build up in your body. The cellular environment is poisoned. Energy declines and degenerative diseases will eventually result.

Toxins in our body come from:

- The thousands of chemicals in our environment, food, and water
- Byproducts of the everyday metabolism of the body

It is not just the smog, pesticides, food additives, alcohol, drinking water, prescription medications, and other external poisons that clog the body. Naturally produced toxins build up as well. The exit route our own toxins take is often not available because:

- They are crowded out of the detoxification system by too many toxins from the environment.
- There is a lack of nutrients available to detoxify them.

The body has an internal garbage removal system that can only handle a lot of debris when it has enough workers. These workers require abundant amounts of vitamins, minerals, and essential fatty acids. RDA amounts are not enough. Our environment and refined food supply have greatly increased our need for cleansing nutrients.

Detoxifying requires nutritional teamwork. Just as a baseball team with great pitching and poor fielding will never win a pennant, a body with high amounts of some detoxifying nutrients and deficiencies of others will not be optimally well. Everything from large amounts of vitamin C to just the right quantities of trace minerals must be present in the right balance. Otherwise, the body cannot keep itself cleansed of toxins and running smoothly. Our nutrient intake will only achieve maximum benefit when optimally balanced.[338]

Enhancing energy requires a two-step approach: detoxifying the body, and rebuilding it with the right nutrients and foods.

Detoxifying

Detoxifying involves:

- Checking for high iron levels through a serum ferritin test and taking appropriate actions to reduce excessive amounts
- Removal—when appropriate—of toxic metals used in dentistry such as mercury fillings and nickel crowns. Some tolerate these toxic materials better than others.
- Limiting our consumption of food grown with pesticides, fungicides, and herbicides
- Eliminating toxic fats such as refined supermarket vegetable oils, margarines, and fried foods
- Quitting smoking and avoiding secondhand smoke
- Improving urban air quality with air filters
- Filtering water to remove fluoride, chlorine and other toxins
- Eliminating coffee, sugar, smoking, and other toxifying stimulants
- Avoiding foods to which one is allergic or sensitive
- Avoiding refined white "enriched" flour products
- Limiting the use of prescription and over-the-counter medications and seeking natural, nontoxic alternatives whenever possible
- Losing weight if necessary
- Cleansing the liver with milk thistle extract and dandelion root
- Using the UltraClear detoxification program (see "Healthy Liver Function" in this chapter)

Rebuilding

Rebuilding involves:

- Consuming vitamins, minerals, essential fatty acids, and amino acids in balanced, optimal amounts
- Receiving small, regular amounts of sunshine[339]
- Eating small amounts of protein throughout the day
- Insuring optimal food digestion and assimilation
- For the acutely ill or those with poor digestion, receiving nutrients intravenously at regular intervals

REAL ENERGY IS THE GOAL

Detoxifying the body to increase energy and health requires time and patience. It takes time to strengthen and tonify a body that has been exhausted from overwork, a lack of rest, and a nutrient-poor diet. Real energy may be slow in returning. Optimal health does not return overnight. The long-term results, however, are worth the time and effort.

Avoid Stimulants

For natural energy to return, all stimulants must be avoided. This includes sugar, stimulant herbs like ephedra, and coffee. All forms of coffee are undesirable, caffeinated or not. It is heavily sprayed with pesticides, and the frequent roasting of coffee creates free-radical-producing substances. All stimulants deplete the body of its energy. They push the body further when it needs rest, nutritional help, detoxification, or attention to deeper metabolic issues. Fatigue is not a coffee deficiency.

Millions of Americans rely on coffee to get them going in the morning.

Coffee is one of the most damaging stimulants because it:
- Depletes valuable minerals needed for energy and bone health
- Stresses adrenal glands, worsening fatigue
- Causes an imbalance in blood sugar
- Toxifies the body with the many pesticides and other harmful chemicals sprayed on the coffee plant
- Raises blood pressure
- Stimulates the flow of stomach acid and produces heartburn
- Interferes with sleep

Unfermented green tea is an excellent alternative to coffee. It has many health-enhancing nutrients. Although green tea is bland-tasting when compared to coffee, putting a cinnamon stick in it or sweetening it with liquid FOS will liven it up. Unfermented green tea has antioxidant, anticancer, and liver-protecting properties.

Exercise

Exercise is essential for abundant energy.

Regular aerobic exercise such as walking and jogging enhances energy by:

- Putting more oxygen in the body. With regular aerobic exercise, the heart pumps more blood and thus delivers more oxygen to the tissues. Increased oxygen levels allow us to burn off more sugars and fats in our cells, thereby raising energy levels.
- Increasing circulation to the brain for more mental energy.
- Increasing tissue response to insulin, which stabilizes mood and blood sugar levels.
- Decreasing free radical production. Exercise helps our cells produce energy more efficiently, producing fewer free radicals that damage tissues and slow us down.
- Stimulating the lymph system to be better able to remove toxins.
- Stimulating improved digestive function so we are better able to absorb energy-releasing nutrients from food.
- Helping to relieve constipation. Constipation fills the body with toxins and causes fatigue.

Exercise is itself a stimulant, and in excess can do more harm than good. Never force yourself to exercise when tired, and do not exercise after a large meal or a meal that is high in fat. Exercising in the right amount should leave you revitalized, not exhausted.

Oxygen

Getting optimal amounts of oxygen in our bodies is one of the most important strategies for maintaining health and energy. This is increasingly difficult to do. The earth's crust contains significantly lower levels of oxygen than it did one hundred years ago. We live mostly indoors, where oxygen is in even shorter supply. For long-term health and energy, do everything possible to receive oxygen in optimal amounts.

Lifestyle habits that deprive us of oxygen include:
- Working in buildings that do not have fresh supplies of air. Large office buildings usually have only recirculated or filtered air. This decreases the amount of oxygen we breathe. Bringing plants to your office can help, especially spider plants. There is no substitute, however, for a fresh supply of air throughout the day. Virgin flaxseed oil as well as supplements of vitamin E and coenzyme Q10 are helpful for those who work in oxygen-depleted surroundings.

- Sleeping at night with closed windows. Even in the winter, try to leave a window open a small crack somewhere in your house. Be sure to adequately ventilate your house once per day, especially during winter months.

Sleep

In this age of technology, we view the human body as yet another piece of indestructible machinery. We think overwork and a lack of rest will not affect its performance. It will. The human body requires a repair period every day during which tissues are fixed, free radicals are neutralized, hormones are manufactured, glands are rejuvenated, and waste products are removed. Without adequate sleep and the right nutrients to effect repairs, the body cannot maintain abundant energy, no matter how many stimulants are used. One of the dangers of using stimulants to compensate for inadequate sleep and poor nutrition is that it deludes one into believing that the body is adequately rested and nourished when it isn't. Overstimulating the body and depriving it of sleep, vitamins, minerals, and essential fatty acids will accelerate aging and cause burnout. Although burnout may arrive suddenly one day, it takes a long time to create. It is the result of years of inadequate nutrition and abuse.

Get enough sleep so that you can awake without an alarm. If you need your alarm clock to wake you up every day, go to bed earlier.

An important hormone known as melatonin is released when we sleep. It is one of the most powerful antioxidants and anti-aging substances produced by the body. Depriving yourself of sleep reduces the amount of time this anti-aging hormone has to restore and rejuvenate the body.

Avoid Sugar

Sugar may give instant energy, but in the long run slows you down. Sugar:

- Depletes B vitamins needed for energy production
- Imbalances blood sugar, causing hypoglycemia and fatigue
- Feeds candida overgrowth in the intestine, which leads to fatigue and depression
- Exhausts the adrenal glands, pancreas and thyroid gland. Glandular exhaustion is a major cause of fatigue.

Avoid Margarine

Stay away from fried foods, margarines, vegetable shortenings, and all baked and snack foods containing partially hydrogenated oils. Use energizing fats like virgin flax and canola oils. Small amounts of butter are also acceptable if you are not allergic to dairy products.

Fried and partially hydrogenated oils need to be avoided because they:

- Interfere with the production of ATP, a substance needed for cellular energy
- Upset cell membrane, liver, and immune system function, which can result in lowered energy levels

Food Allergies

Avoid foods that you may be allergic to. It is often difficult to determine which foods may be causing problems, but it is a very important strategy for improving energy levels. The most common allergenic foods are wheat, dairy products, citrus fruits, and soy products. Often the food you love and eat most frequently is the one you are most sensitive to. The best way to find out whether your energy level is affected by a food is to eliminate that food from your diet and note whether you feel a difference in your energy and well-being. After two weeks, add the food back to your diet. If you note a return of lower energy levels, eat that food as infrequently as possible.

Healthy Liver Function

The liver is one of the most important organs for helping to maintain good energy levels. The liver rids the body of toxins, cleans the blood, and helps maintain a state of hormonal balance. Adequate protein along with optimal vitamin and mineral intake will help keep your liver functioning well. Plenty of spring or distilled water and freshly prepared vegetable juices — especially tomato juice — are also energizing through their ability to stimulate optimal liver function.

Smog, chemicals from copiers and other office machines, pesticides on produce, oral contraceptives, medications, alcohol, and secondhand smoke all slow the liver down. One of the most powerful supplements to help the liver to strengthen and detoxify itself is standardized milk thistle extract. It has been extensively studied for its ability to protect and repair the liver.

The UltraClear program developed by Dr. Jeffrey Bland is a state-of-the-art detoxifying program that cleanses the liver of toxic material. It is hypoallergenic, nutritionally balanced, and has yielded remarkable results in patients whose diseases were caused or worsened by their inability to remove cellular garbage. It is highly recommended for anyone with energy problems or ailments related to inadequate cellular detoxification. This includes food allergies, chemical sensitivities, chronic fatigue, toxic-metal-induced hypertension, and a range of other degenerative diseases. It is must be done under the supervision of a health professional.

Skeletal Alignment

Nerves that transmit signals to our body must not be impeded by a poorly aligned spinal column. If the spine is out of line, it decreases the amount of information that nerve cells transmit to the rest of the body. A decrease in health and energy results. Practitioners such as chiropractors and osteopaths can correct these "subluxations" or misalignments in the spine. An aligned skeletal system is literally the backbone of abundant energy.

Environmental Factors

Some develop environmental allergies to chemicals given off by paint, kitchen floors, newsprint, or any one of the thousands of chemicals that assault us daily. In susceptible people, this can lead to depression, fatigue, and poor immune function. Electromagnetic radiation from power lines, computer monitors, television, and other sources can also lead to fatigue. When buying a computer, insist on a monitor that meets low radiation standards.

Candida Albicans

Candida albicans is a yeast normally present in the intestinal tract in small amounts. When it transforms into its fungal form and overgrows, energy and mood levels go down. Such an overgrowth is best treated with a low-carbohydrate, sugar-free diet that includes beneficial bacteria such as bifidobacterium. Immune-boosting nutrients such as zinc, vitamin C, vitamin E, and essential fatty acids are also helpful. Although candida occurs most frequently in women, both sexes are capable of succumbing to an overgrowth.

SUMMING UP

There are no shortcuts to optimal energy. You must pursue health on every level to have abundant energy throughout your life. And it can often take time and patience to allow real energy levels to return. There are, however, beneficial supplements that can accelerate our progression toward a state of more optimal health and energy. These nutrients are often the key, as we shall see, for helping increase the body's ability to turn food into energy at a more efficient rate.

CHAPTER 22

Energy-Enhancing Nutrients

TWENTY MINUTES AFTER YOU EAT a banana, your heart, brain, and skeletal muscles are using it as a source of power. This remarkable process of turning food into energy confounds chemistry students with its complexity. Yet all you need to know is that if you have the right nutrients, it will happen effortlessly. If you don't, it won't. One missing vitamin, mineral, or other nutrient will slow you down.

There are many ways nutrients keep us energetic. Nutrients combat fatigue by neutralizing free radicals that are given off by the body as a part of everyday metabolism. Free radicals interfere with your metabolism, and the right nutrients neutralize them. Vitamins and minerals are needed by the glandular system for the creation of energy-releasing hormones. A wide range of nutrients is needed to keep the immune system strong so that we will not be slowed down by a cold or other illness.

Not all supplements that enhance energy do so in a way that is health-promoting. Stimulant herbs such as ephedra should only be used for short periods of time. Vitamins, minerals, essential fats, and tonic herbs such as ginseng, schizandra, dandelion root, and others are safe and beneficial as long-term energy aids.

Also beneficial are nonvitamin nutrients such as CoQ10, carnitine, and dimethylglycine (DMG). By understanding which nutrients are helpful, we can help our bodies build stamina and immune and organ function, and generate a state of optimal health from which energy freely flows.

Energizing nutrients come in three varieties: nutrients, which help the body to combust food; tonics, which help build up body systems over time and strengthen the glands; and stimulants, which should be avoided, for they push the body too far and burn it out.

ENERGIZING NUTRIENTS

The body burns food the same way a car explodes gasoline—a little at a time, under very controlled conditions, and in a way that will not harm surrounding structures. Nutrients are the spark plugs that help us to derive energy from the food we combust. If we are missing any nutrients, we will be less able to get energy from the food we eat. This can cause low levels of energy, weight gain, and food cravings.

Just as sparks fly out of a fireplace when logs are burned, free radicals emanate from our cells as food is combusted. These free radicals must be neutralized if energy levels are to remain high. That is why antioxidants such as vitamin C, vitamin E, and beta-carotene are important for maintaining good energy levels under stress. Free radicals in excess slow us down.

B complex. B complex vitamins are needed in different amounts by different people. Many vitamin preparations contain up to 100 milligrams of the B complex. Those with slow metabolisms or with blood sugar problems find this amount helpful. Pantothenic acid (B_5) is particularly important for maintaining high energy levels in times of stress.

Vitamin E. Without enough vitamin E, red blood cell membranes disintegrate and these cells lose their oxygen-carrying hemoglobin. When this happens, vitamin-E-deficient anemias can develop. Fewer red blood cells means the body has a harder time bringing oxygen to tissues. This results in lower energy levels, a slower metabolism, and difficulty losing weight.[340] Vitamin B_6, copper, folic acid, and B_{12} are also needed to make sure that red blood cells are strong and healthy.

Iron. Iron is the most important mineral for the health of red blood cells and is of critical importance for maintaining energy levels. Menstruating and pregnant women are often at risk of having low levels of iron. They often benefit from supplementation. This is especially true for women who avoid meat or who experience heavy periods. Before taking iron, have your iron levels checked by your physician with a blood test known as serum ferritin. Otherwise, you may be giving

your body iron that it does not need. This will only worsen
your fatigue.

Iron has been overprescribed for fatigue, especially for
men, who are rarely deficient. For years, iron was viewed as a
universally beneficial tonic. Recent research has shown that
when iron is taken in excess, it is stored in various organs and
tissues in the body, increasing the risk for cancer, heart disease, diabetes, and aging. Unfortunately, the chief symptom of
iron overload is the same as that of deficiency: fatigue.

Potassium. This is an extremely important mineral for
optimal energy levels. Before you buy an expensive potassium
elixir, start eating plenty of steamed vegetables like broccoli
and carrots. Virtually all whole, unprocessed foods have significant amounts of potassium. Change your diet to one of only
whole, unrefined foods. Freshly prepared juices from carrots,
leafy greens, and other fruits and vegetables are a very good
way to get plenty of energizing potassium. Just don't overdo the
fruit juices, for their high sugar content can slow you down.

Magnesium. Magnesium is another critical mineral needed
for energy production. Few of us get in optimal amounts. Too
much calcium with a corresponding lack of magnesium can
create fatigue. While calcium is needed for healthy bones, it
must be balanced with magnesium and other minerals in the
diet or energy levels will decline.

Zinc. Critical to proper energy production, zinc is quickly
depleted by stress, whether physical or emotional. A lack of
zinc will make it difficult for you to keep blood sugar balanced
or for you to digest food well. It can also impair mental function
and weaken your immune system.

Flax oil. Flax oil helps give you the calm, even energy you
need to combat stress. It is one of the most important foods to
keep the nervous system well nourished. Make sure that the
flax oil you buy comes in a black, opaque plastic container in
the refrigerated section of your health food store. Only use it in
recipes that do not involve heat. One to three tablespoons per
day is the amount most find helpful.

GLA. Essential fats such as GLA have been shown to help
your body make more ATP, the energy currency of the cell. The
more ATP you make, the more energetic you will be. Make sure
that you take enough, however, if you are trying to increase
energy levels. You must get at least 500 milligrams of GLA to
see any effect. This amount of GLA is found in two 1,000-

milligram capsules of borage oil capsules or eleven capsules of evening primrose oil. Essential fatty acids exert their benefits more effectively when total fat intake is kept to no more than 30% of total calories.

L-Carnitine. L-Carnitine is a nutrient that acts like a fork-lift, carrying fatty acids to the part of the cell where they are transformed into energy. Carnitine is helpful in promoting weight   loss and energy production. Our bodies make small amounts of L-Carnitine. Optimal levels are available only through supplementation. Since Carnitine is found predominantly in animal products such as red meat, vegetarians may have a special need to supplement. Most find 250–1,000 milligrams per day helpful.

CoEnzyme Q10. Before you can spend money in France, you have to change it into francs. Before you can turn food into energy, you have to first change the sugars and starches you eat into the energy currency of the cell, called ATP. To maximize your ability to turn food into ATP, you need optimal levels of many nutrients, especially CoQ10. CoQ10 is a substance manufactured by the body in small amounts, not optimal amounts, and less as we age.

Supplements of CoQ10 have been shown to help increase energy levels, lower blood pressure, promote weight loss, enhance gum health, and stimulate immune function. CoQ10 strengthens the heart and acts as the first nutritional line of defense against heart disease by protecting cholesterol from sticking to arteries. Typical supplemental doses range between 25 and 100 milligrams per day.

Tonics

There are many products that help nourish the body and gradually build energy levels. They may give instant increases in energy. Usually, however, they must be taken for a period of time before results are seen.

Ginseng is a name used to cover a family of plants that are the best-studied and most effective herbal tonics in the world. There are many types of ginseng on the market, and all have been shown to be effective for helping build energy levels gradually and without a stimulant effect. Siberian ginseng (*Eleutherococcus senticosus*), American ginseng (*Panax quinquefolius*), and Korean ginseng (*Panax ginseng*) are three of the best known. A knowledgeable herbalist can help you determine which kind is right for you.

Thousands of studies have demonstrated the benefits of ginseng. Ginseng helps to detoxify the body of pollution that can slow the body down. It helps support the adrenal glands, which help us maintain balanced energy levels. Ginseng has also been shown to help keep blood sugar and blood pressure in normal ranges. It rebalances the body in innumerable ways. It may be one of the most valuable substances to help the body combat the damaging effects of stress.

As our knowledge of ginseng expands, so does demand for it. Ginseng can be expensive. Make sure you are getting the real thing. The best way to be sure you will get the full effects of ginseng is to buy from a manufacturer who lists "standardized ginseng extract" on the label.

Other tonics that are beneficial include schizandra, gotu kola, dandelion root, and licorice. All of these botanicals have been researched for their ability to enhance the function of the body systems that maintain our energy levels.

Royal jelly is a highly concentrated food made by worker bees to feed the queen bee. It is the richest natural source for pantothenic acid, a B vitamin needed for energy production and stress management. Half of the dry weight of royal jelly is easily assimilated protein.[341] It is also rich in other B vitamins, many minerals, and contains a wide variety of unique compounds. Royal jelly is increasingly popular as a supplement for those who want to maximize their energy levels, and may offer a wide variety of other benefits as well. For example, royal jelly has also been found to contain insulinlike actions that may be of benefit to diabetics.[342]

Unique antibacterial substances have also been found in royal jelly, including the protein Royalisin and the fatty acid known as 10-HDA. Whole royal jelly itself has ten times the disinfectant power of just one of these compounds. Researchers feel the major antimicrobial compounds in royal jelly have yet to be identified.[343, 344]

According to animal studies, 10-HDA in royal jelly also has powerful antitumor activity. Both unprocessed royal jelly and 10-HDA were studied over a two-year period with two thousand mice. All of the mice receiving injections of tumor cells plus royal jelly or 10-HDA remained alive and healthy for more than twelve months. The sister mice, which received the same number of tumor cells without royal jelly, all died within twelve days. Further trials of 10-HDA and royal jelly in cancer patients are warranted.[345]

For maximum benefit, I recommend royal jelly that has not been processed or freeze-dried. This ensures that the proteins and delicate fatty acids are intact.

Stimulants

Although stimulants may be useful in the short term for needed energy or other nutritional benefit, in the long term they can stress the body and burn it out even further. When the body is tired, it does not want to be whipped into doing more, which is exactly what stimulant herbs will do. It is far better to use standardized ginsengs that build energy slowly than to abuse the body further.

Ephedra, which is also known as **ma huang**, has the oldest recorded use of any herbal product. Chinese writings mention it over five thousand years ago. It is a stimulant used by many for increased mental alertness and energy, and may also provide symptomatic relief for sinus congestion. This herb, especially in tincture form, should be used with caution because it is an adrenal stimulant that can be overused and become addictive. Prolonged use of ephedra, kola nut, and other stimulant herbs will only weaken the body and deprive us of what we hoped they would give us: energy.

CHAPTER 23

Nutrition for Healthy Skin

THE MOST POWERFUL STRATEGY YOU can employ to get vibrant skin is to pursue optimal health. Your skin doesn't lie. Makeup, natural cleansing agents, and spa treatments can help, but they will never cover up the effects of missing nutrients and toxic foods. Like any other part of your body, your skin requires an abundant supply of nutrients to look and feel its best. If you have been good to your body, your skin will show it.

Skin requires the right kind of fatty acids, vitamins, and minerals. These nutrients take time to reach the skin when we change and improve our diet. It may be weeks or even months before the rewards of good nutrition become apparent in our skin. Yet patience is rewarded. The skin is highly responsive to optimal nutrition. Almost every skin problem can be helped through eating a more health-promoting diet.

STRATEGIES FOR HEALTHY SKIN

Avoid margarine and all foods that contain hydrogenated oils. Hydrogenated oils have many negative effects on the skin, which gives you an idea of what they do to the rest of your body. Hydrogenated oils interfere with hormones known as prostaglandins that keep skin healthy. Teens eat a lot of margarine, especially in the prepackaged cookies, baked goods, chips, and other junk foods in the adolescent diet. Avoid anything that contains these toxic fats if you want healthy skin.

Eliminate fried foods. This includes potato chips, fried pies and all deep fried dishes. These highly heated fats have negative effects on overall wellness and skin health.

Promote Intestinal Health. Fiber-rich foods and beneficial bacteria are both essential for healthy skin. A lack of fiber leads to constipation, which causes toxins to circulate throughout the body and come out through the skin. Unfriendly bacteria in the GI tract increase the amount of garbage the liver has to detoxify, and an unhealthy liver will lead to decreased skin health. Supplements of friendly bacteria such as acidophilus, bifidobacterium, and bulgaricus promote skin health by detoxifying the GI tract and enhancing nutrient absorption. Candida albicans overgrowth, parasites, and other GI disorders must be ruled out when any skin problems do not respond to changes in diet and nutrient intake.

Promote liver health. The liver and the skin are both organs of detoxification. If the liver is not doing a good job getting rid of toxic material, more toxins will come out through the skin, decreasing skin quality. That is why a healthy liver is critical for skin health. The UltraClear detoxification program available through your nutritionist or nutritionally oriented health care practitioner is one of the best ways to cleanse the liver and improve the quality of the skin. Standardized milk thistle extract and dandelion root are also very useful for helping improve liver health.

Don't smoke. Smoking is one of the most damaging things you can do to your skin. Avoid smoke-filled bars and ask your friends who smoke not to do it around you.

Exercise and get adequate rest. Both are very important for healthy skin.

SUPPLEMENTS FOR HEALTHY SKIN

Vitamin C, both taken as a supplement and applied topically, is one of the most important nutrients for skin health and protection. It should be one of the main ingredients in sunscreen formulas. Exposure to UV radiation destroys two thirds of the vitamin C in skin. Topically applied vitamin C inhibits radiation damage from the sun. It also slows the development of wrinkles and premature aging of the skin.[346, 347] Sunscreens with vitamin C can make spending time in the sun a much safer activity.[348]

Magnesium is one of the most important nutrients for beautiful skin. It may be especially helpful along with the B complex and antioxidant nutrients in preventing wrinkles.

According to the USDA, most Americans do not get enough of this nutrient. Helpful supplemental amounts: 400–600 milligrams per day of magnesium oxide or citrate. Epsom salt baths are another way to get more magnesium in the body.

Zinc is extremely important for healthy skin. Countless studies show most Americans do not get enough zinc. Zinc is needed for the production of new healthy skin cells. Red meat, seafood, oysters, and nuts and seeds are some of the few foods that contain zinc. Few eat these foods every day.

Zinc has been found especially useful in the treatment of acne. Useful amounts of zinc for skin problems are 25–50 milligrams zinc as zinc picolinate per day. Long-term zinc supplementing should be balanced with copper.[349]

Water is very important for skin health. Drink 6 to 8 glasses per day. Distilled or spring water or the water in freshly made vegetable juices is best.

Essential Fats are extremely important for the skin. Flaxseed oil, a member of the omega-3 family of fats, is the ideal salad oil. Virgin canola oil is also very valuable. These oils should be kept refrigerated. Flax oil should only be used in nonheat recipes. One to two tablespoons of these oils per day is usually best. Many people find flax oil helps their skin acquire a velvety smoothness.

EPA is an essential fatty acid found in fish oils and cold-water fish, especially salmon, sardines, and mackerel. Many find EPA helpful in rebalancing the health of their skin. Countless studies show EPA's anti-inflammatory effect. EPA is a delicate oil and needs to be taken with vitamin E so that it does not oxidize in the body.

GLA is an essential fatty acid and an extraordinary food for the skin. It lubricates the skin, making it remarkably supple and smooth. GLA is made by the body in small amounts. Growing older, low thyroid function, eating hydrogenated oils, consuming fried foods and sugar, or underconsuming magnesium, zinc, vitamin C, B3, and B_6 will all decrease the body's ability to make GLA. GLA is found in evening primrose and borage oil supplements.

SKIN AND THE SUN

The ozone layer that protects our skin from damaging UV radiation is thinning. This is one of the reasons skin cancer rates are rising every year. Overconsumption of refined omega-6 fats like corn oil, safflower oil, and sunflower oil increase risk of skin cancer. Toxic chemicals in many tanning lotions also may damage the skin when mixed with free-radical-producing sunlight. Many of the toxins in our environment and food supply may damage the skin as they are excreted through the skin in the presence of sunlight. All of these factors must be avoided by those who have to spend significant amounts of time in the sun. Choose sunscreens and tanning lotions that are rich in antioxidants and as low in synthetic chemicals as possible.

Increase your intake of the antioxidants vitamin A, C, E, beta-carotene, B_2, zinc, selenium, taurine, and NAC when you go in the sun, especially if you tend to sunburn. Take all antioxidants rather than just one or two of them. A balanced intake is much more protective. It is easily obtained by using any of the high-quality antioxidant formulations available. Many studies have shown that antioxidants may be a very important strategy for preventing skin cancer.[350]

Don't take EPA, GLA, or flax oil in significant quantities if you spend a great deal of time in the sun. These delicate oils can make your skin sensitive to sunlight.

Tanning may look healthy, but a tan is a protective mechanism in reaction to skin damage. Don't completely avoid the sun, but keep sun exposure to a minimum. Always wear sunglasses that filter out all UV rays.

SKIN PROBLEMS

Acne. When the teenage body begins to mature, it has to decide how to ration the small amounts of zinc and essential fatty acids it is given through the typical junk food diet. Should it use them to nourish the many maturing organs, particularly the gonads, or should it use them to promote skin health? The body's wisdom shunts them to the internal organs, and the skin suffers.

Acne is not an inevitable part of growing up. If optimal amounts of zinc and essential fatty acids were present, such rationing would not be necessary, and psychologically devastating teenage acne could be avoided. This most common form of acne, *acne vulgaris*, responds very well to optimal nutrition. Though it usually occurs during adolescence, it can occur any time hormones, stress, missing nutrients, and intestinal problems combine to create havoc for the skin. Antibiotics may improve symptoms initially, but in the long run will worsen the condition by causing a deterioration of the health of the intestinal tract.[351]

Foods that clog the liver, such as fried foods, hydrogenated oils, and alcohol, must be avoided. Sugar and refined carbohydrates such as white bread should also be eliminated. Sugar feeds unfriendly bacteria that negatively affect the skin and liver, and depletes many nutrients needed for skin health.

Nutrients that have been found to be beneficial for acne sufferers include vitamin A, vitamin E, folic acid, B_6, zinc, and selenium. Chromium may be of particular importance for those with acne. Acne may be caused or worsened by poor tissue response to insulin. Chromium picolinate improves insulin metabolism. Check also for food sensitivities, especially to foods such as wheat and dairy. Iron-fortified foods should be avoided. Synthetic iron destroys vitamin E and essential fatty acids.

Combination Skin. Skin that is part dry, part oily is caused by eating margarine, hydrogenated oils, fried and processed foods. GLA and flax oil are very helpful at restoring the balance of essential fatty acids and eliminating combination skin. Minerals such as zinc and magnesium are also helpful.

Eczema. Eliminating foods such as wheat and dairy products for a month is recommended to see if a sensitivity exists that may cause or exacerbate eczema. Other foods, such as potatoes, chocolate, eggs, and soy products, may also cause problems. If food allergy testing is unavailable, pick one food to avoid for a two-week period and watch for improvement. Helpful supplements for eczema include GLA, digestive enzymes, vitamins A, C, E, and B complex, zinc, and flaxseed oil.

Psoriasis. This is a condition in which skin cells replicate too quickly, giving the skin a scaly appearance. It has a variety of causes, including nutritional deficiencies, food sensitivities, and stress. Improving digestion and liver function, replacing missing essential fatty acids, and correcting mineral deficiencies are helpful. It is important to increase fiber content of the diet and consume leafy greens, which help detoxify the bowel. Folic acid, vitamins A, C, and E, vitamin B_{12} injections, zinc, selenium, and EPA benefit those with psoriasis. Small amounts of sunlight have also been found to be helpful.

SUMMING UP

- Skin problems respond well to optimal nutrition.
- Healthy skin requires a wide array of nutrients, healthy liver function, good digestion and assimilation of nutrients, and abundant amounts of beneficial bacteria in the intestinal tract.
- Avoid hydrogenated oils, fried foods, refined supermarket oils, sugar, white flour products, and alcohol.
- GLA, flax oil, and zinc are particularly helpful.
- Drink plenty of water.
- Small amounts of sun are beneficial; too much is damaging.
- Healthy skin requires adequate sleep and regular exercise.

CHAPTER 24

Maximizing Hair Health

MANY HAIR PROBLEMS ARE GENETIC and hormonal, and outside the reach of nutrition. Yet significant improvement in hair quality is often seen by improving the diet and lifestyle and optimizing intake of certain nutrients.

AVOID SUGAR

One of the most important strategies for keeping the hair you have is to avoid sugar. If you cannot get rid of your sugar cravings, supplement with zinc and chromium and eat regular amounts of protein throughout the day.

EAT ENOUGH PROTEIN

Your hair is protein. If you do not eat enough, you may experience hair loss. Low protein diets are a common cause of hair loss, easily reversed by consuming normal amounts. Sulfur-rich foods such as eggs and other high-quality protein foods are very beneficial for the hair. Most people require at least two 4-ounce servings of protein per day. Supplements of predigested protein help many people with thinning hair. This suggests that poor digestion and inadequate protein intake are often present.

GOOD CIRCULATION

Good circulation is needed to feed the hair. All of the nutrients that build healthy red blood cells and keep arteries clear are necessary: antioxidants, essential fatty acids, vitamins B_6, folic acid, B_{12}, and adequate iron. Exercise is also important.

AVOID CAFFEINATED BEVERAGES

The caffeine in coffee and tea depletes the body of minerals needed to grow healthy hair. It also causes the body to lose water that it needs to help feed the hair. Drink six to eight glasses of spring or distilled water per day. Natural herbal iced tea mixes available at health food stores can liven up the taste of water. These natural drinks also contain trace minerals valuable to hair.

GOOD DIGESTION

If you are not digesting your food well, your body will not get the protein and minerals it needs to make healthy-looking hair. Many people have insufficient stomach acid, poor pancreatic function, and an overstressed GI tract from years of poor eating habits, antacid abuse, and overeating. For this reason it may be beneficial to use digestive supplements. Digestive enzymes should always be taken with meals. Those with digestive ailments such as ulcers should only take digestive aids under the supervision of a health professional.

VITAMINS

Vitamin A is a very important nutrient for the hair. Hair cannot be shiny and healthy without it. Most of us derive vitamin A from beta-carotene in produce, which must in turn be converted by the body into vitamin A. Adequate thyroid function is necessary to convert beta-carotene into vitamin A. If your thyroid is not functioning adequately, this conversion won't happen efficiently. If you have low thyroid function and have poor-quality hair, you may benefit from 10,000 to 25,000 IUs per day of vitamin A palmitate. Pregnant women should take no more than 8,000 IUs per day, and only under the guidance of a physician.

The B complex vitamins, particularly folic acid, B_{12}, and pantothenic acid, are all needed for healthy hair. Inositol may also be helpful. Anecdotally, biotin at doses of 5 milligrams per day or more has also produced noticeable improvement in hair quality in some.

MINERALS

Minerals that are needed for healthy hair include copper, selenium, iron, and zinc. Body levels of these minerals should be balanced. Too much iron will destroy vitamin E. Excessive copper will make it difficult for hair to respond to a permanent. Hair analysis, while more indicative of body mineral levels than the specific health of the hair, is an excellent way to help determine which minerals may be present in excess. Testing is recommended so that individual needs can be met.

Silica is a trace mineral that many have found helpful in improving the health of their hair and nails. Extracts of spring horsetail may be the best way to add silica to the diet. Don't confuse silica with silicone, which is used in breast implants.

NAC

N-Acetyl Cysteine is not only one of the most valuable antioxidant nutrients. It also supplies sulfur needed for hair health. Do not take hair formulas that contain L-Cysteine—it is too unstable and oxidizes readily. NAC offers much more benefit. It should be taken on an empty stomach for maximum absorption. Diabetics should avoid NAC. Cysteine in any form can block insulin receptors on cell membranes.

SPICES

Cayenne (red pepper powder) and ginger are used by many in an effort to help stimulate circulation to the scalp. There are no studies to show whether this is effective, but adding small amounts of these spices to your shampoo is harmless. Keep this stinging mixture out of your eyes.

HORMONAL FACTORS

Thyroid insufficiency can often lead to the loss or thinning of hair. An imbalance in other hormones can also lead to facial hair in women. These issues are best discussed with your physician or endocrinologist.

MALE PATTERN BALDNESS

Male hormones are at the root of this problem. It cannot be reversed with nutrition. Hair loss may be slowed, however, through an optimal intake of nutrients, avoiding sugar, and ensuring good circulation and adequate protein digestion.

Can Saw Palmetto Help?

An excessive amount of a testosterone derivative known as dihydrotestosterone may be responsible for the hair loss of male pattern baldness. Topical treatments of testosterone have been shown to slow male pattern baldness by halting the formation of dihydrotestosterone.[352] High-quality standardized extracts of the saw palmetto plant have also been found to inhibit the formation of dihydrotestosterone. Whether taking saw palmetto supplements will slow the progression of male pattern baldness remains to be seen.

Tridax Procumbens

Tridax procumbens is a plant that grows in India and is used in hair tonics in that country. Preliminary animal studies demonstrate that both topical treatment and oral use of this plant stimulate hair growth in albino rats. Indian Ayruvedic medicine has long used Tridax for hair problems. More studies are needed to see if it can promote human hair growth.[353]

CHEMOTHERAPY AND HAIR LOSS

Dr. Robert Cathcart is one of the country's best-known physicians specializing in the use of high-dose vitamin C for a variety of conditions. He has found that if enough vitamin C is consumed orally by cancer patients, hair loss caused by chemotherapy can be eliminated. The dose for this effect is high—between 10 and 50 grams per day in divided doses, or until bowel tolerance is reached. It should be taken with the guidance of a nutritionally oriented physician. Studies have shown that high doses of vitamin C do not blunt the cancer-killing effect of chemotherapy: They enhance its effectiveness.

SUMMING UP

- Consume adequate amounts of protein every day.
- Avoid all sugars. Even too much dried fruit or fruit juice adversely affects hair.
- Take supplemental vitamins and minerals.

- Avoid caffeinated beverages.
- Work with a health professional who can assess your hormonal balance, digestive function, and circulation.
- Exercise frequently.
- Incorporate stress management techniques into your life.

CHAPTER 25

Nutrition and Aging

O LDER ADULTS NEED OPTIMAL NUTRITION to help compensate
for the decreased function of their bodies and their
increased susceptibility to disease. As we age, our
bodies no longer digest, assimilate and metabolize food as well
as they to. They need a greatly increased intake of virtually all
essential nutrients.

If you are on prescription or over-the-counter medications,
work with your physician to keep the number to a minimum.
Drugs often decrease the functional ability of the liver and put
stress on other organs like the kidneys. If you have high blood
pressure, high cholesterol, or digestive problems, work with
your physician and a nutritionist to help rebalance your body
through natural means. Drugs play a valuable role in treating
acute conditions but are needlessly overused. Be assertive.
Change physicians if necessary and find one who understands
the value of nutrition. Most doctors prefer to keep you on a
medication because they lack both the time and knowledge to
offer you natural solutions.

BASIC NUTRITION FOR OLDER ADULTS

Older people need fewer calories because they have less muscle
mass and a slower metabolism. While older people need fewer
calories, their need for protein remains the same and their need
for many vitamins, minerals, and essential fatty acids increases.
As we age, we need to eat foods that are higher in nutrients. Junk
foods at any age are undesirable, but are especially so for seniors,
who need to get more nutrients out of less food.

Forty percent of people age 51 and older do not eat enough. Two out of every five seniors eat less than two thirds of their recommended caloric intake. This lowered food intake is one of the causes for the widespread nutritional deficiencies among the elderly. It may be caused or worsened by zinc deficiency. When the body lacks zinc, appetite decreases and a vicious circle of undernutrition begins.

Older adults have low levels of nutrients because:

- 40% of them do not eat enough
- They have a decreased ability to digest, absorb, and metabolize nutrients
- Their medications deplete nutrients
- The activity of their defensive enzymes decreases, causing them to use up their antioxidant nutrients more quickly

The suboptimal levels of vitamins and minerals found in older adults can cause dangerously depressed immune function, acceleration of existing diseases, dementia, and other problems. For these and other reasons, high-quality and easily absorbed supplements are essential.[354, 355]

Activated Fatty Acids

As we age, the activity of the enzymes that activate essential fatty acids decreases. Seniors often benefit from already-activated essential fatty acids such as GLA (gamma-linolenic acid) and EPA (eicosapentaenoic acid), found in foods and supplements. GLA is found in few foods but can be easily acquired through supplements of evening primrose oil and borage oil. EPA is found in cold water fish such as sardines, mackerel, salmon, and albacore tuna.

Multivitamins for Older Adults

Most of the multivitamins taken by seniors are low in quality and not balanced for their unique needs. Make sure that your multivitamin does not contain vitamin D, iron, or high amounts of copper unless you are deficient in them.

A double-blind study of ninety-six healthy elderly people showed that by taking a multivitamin, they could cut their incidence of infectious disease in half. Their immune function was markedly enhanced by the multivitamin used in this study even though it contained only RDA levels for most nutrients. Imagine what optimal levels of nutrients could do.[356]

Vitamin A. Vitamin A has been found to protect those who have suffered a stroke. Those with higher levels of vitamin A were found to recover more quickly and were less likely to die. Vitamin A prevents damage to neurons that occurs when oxygen supply to the brain is cut off.[357]

B Vitamins. A recent study from Belgium demonstrated that B_6, B_{12}, and folic acid are often deficient in the elderly. Normal blood tests did not detect the deficiencies. They were only discovered when ornate cellular tests were done. Another recent study showed that seniors who ate more than the RDA for B_1 were still deficient in its metabolically active form—another sign that RDA levels are not enough. Seniors simply do not metabolize vitamins the way younger people do, and need higher amounts.[358] Supplements that contain 50 milligrams of the B complex, 800 micrograms of folic acid, and 100 micrograms of B_{12} can help meet these needs.[359, 360]

Niacin. Vitamin B_3 is an extremely important antisenility nutrient. The research of Dr. Abram Hoffer and others has shown that niacin can prevent and even reverse many of the symptoms of senility. Doses as little as 100 milligrams per day can be effective as a preventive measure. Larger supervised doses are needed for those who exhibit signs of senility. Niacin may cause a harmless flushing reaction when first taken. Niacin is not recommended for those with unstable heart conditions or diabetes. The only time-released, nonflushing form that is recommended is inositol hexanicotinate.

Vitamin B_6. The amount of B_6 needed for optimal immune function is far greater than the current RDA. This is especially true for the elderly, in whom low levels of B_6 have been found to cause a significant decrease in immunity.[361]

Vitamin B_{12}. B_{12} deficiency is common in the elderly. Groups of elderly subjects who tested lowest in B_{12} and folic acid also had the poorest cognitive function scores.[362] Those who are fifty-five years and older have reduced B_{12} absorption, and even less is absorbed as one grows older.[363] Many of the elderly with dementia and confusion have been found to improve with B_{12} injections. B_{12} may be an essential supplement for those age 60 and older, especially those with cognitive difficulties. Low levels of folic acid can also contribute to dementia.[364]

Vitamin E. In a recent study, thirty-two healthy men and women over age sixty were given 800 milligrams per day of vitamin E. This optimal dose of vitamin E boosted their immune function considerably. No one in this study had a "deficiency" of vitamin E. This study clearly demonstrated vitamin E should be thought of as a natural immune-boosting agent regardless of whether one is deficient. Generous intakes of virtually all nutrients — not just vitamin E — should be a routine preventive measure with all senior citizens. They should be as universally recommended as flu shots.[365, 366]

Vitamin C and Beta-Carotene. These are protective nutrients that older adults need to get more of. Studies have shown that as we age, we are often deficient in these nutrients. They both lower the risk of cancer in people over seventy. They are also helpful for preventing heart disease and cataracts.[367, 368]

Magnesium. The elderly are almost always in need of magnesium due to decreased absorption, poor intake, and the use of magnesium-depleting medications such as diuretics. Doses of up to 1,000 milligrams per day have been used successfully in improving the symptoms of dementia. Magnesium is an important nutrient that keeps aluminum from concentrating in the brain. It may be one of the most important nutrients for the prevention of Alzheimer's disease.[369]

Iron. Iron is a double-edged sword. Many older adults lack iron. The fortification of food with iron, however, along with the ubiquitous presence of 18 milligrams of it in virtually every multivitamin, poses the very real danger of getting too much. While iron is needed to maintain good circulation and is important for optimal brain function, excess iron leads to heart disease and cancer.[370] To determine your iron needs, have your physician perform a serum ferritin test. As a general rule of thumb, avoid all iron supplements and fortified foods. If you are given an iron supplement to rectify iron-poor blood, be tested regularly to see if you should continue taking it.

Zinc. Zinc is deficient in up to 95% of the senior citizen population. It is also universally deficient in the elderly hospitalized population.[371] This has staggering implications. Many of the problems that face the older adults, including arthritis, depression, macular degeneration, poor eating habits and taste perception, and poor immune function, are caused or worsened by zinc deficiency. Decreased secretion of stomach acid, widespread in the elderly, will lessen absorption of zinc and other minerals. Zinc supplements of at least 15 milligrams are recommended for adults over age sixty, and should be balanced with 1 milligram of copper.[372, 373, 374]

Selenium. Selenium is an important trace mineral for older adults. Deficiency is common. Selenium has been found to boost immune function significantly in the elderly. It has many other benefits, such as protecting the heart, arteries, eyes, and liver, and should be a part of every senior's supplement program.[375]

Ginkgo. Ginkgo is an herbal preparation made from the maidenhair tree. It is one of the most valuable products ever developed for maintaining and enhancing brain health. It has been used in Chinese medicine for over five thousand years. There are approximately one hundred thousand practitioners worldwide who each year use over ten million prescriptions of an extract of ginkgo biloba with their patients to enhance vascular and cerebral circulation. Over forty double-blind placebo-controlled studies have shown ginkgo to be a powerful antioxidant and liver protector. It also enhances circulation to the brain and heart.[376]

In a six month double-blind placebo-controlled study of thirty-one patients in their fifties with mild to moderate memory loss, a supplement of 40 milligrams of gingko 24% standardized extract was given three times per day. The ginkgo was shown to improve cognitive function significantly without any side effects.[377, 378] Make sure you use the standardized extracts of ginkgo. They are the most studied preparations.[379]

CATARACTS: A PREVENTABLE EPIDEMIC

Cataracts affect four hundred thousand Americans annually. Cataracts cloud the lens of the eye. Vision can decline in varying degrees from a mild loss of sight to blindness. The increase in the incidence of cataracts is faster than that of any other ailment. Many believe that the cause of this dramatic increase in cataracts is the thinning of the ozone layer, a protective shield that, until recently, gave our eyes enough protection against damaging UV radiation.

Keep Sun Exposure to a Minimum
Never look directly into the sun. Sunglasses that protect against all forms of ultraviolet light—both UVA and UVB—should always be worn when outside, even on cloudy days.

Optimize Antioxidant Intake
Those with cataracts have lower levels of antioxidant nutrients such as vitamin E and beta-carotene.[380] Vitamins B_2, C, and E, beta-carotene, zinc, and selenium slow cataract progression.[381] Researchers at the USDA Human Research Center suggest the minimum dose of vitamin C needed to prevent cataracts is 800 milligrams per day.[382, 383] Taurine is an amino acid that is one of the most important antioxidants in the eye.[384, 385] It is useful for the treatment of macular degeneration and to protect the eye from free radical damage. Taurine deficiency will increase damage to the retina.[386, 387]

Eat plenty of fruits and vegetables and take antioxidants for maximum eye protection. Health food stores offer many well-designed eye-protecting formulas. They are highly recommended for seniors, lifeguards, and anyone at increased risk to light damage to their eyes.

Digestive Problems
Digestive problems are common in those over age sixty. Half the population over age sixty does not make enough stomach acid to digest their food adequately. All digestive secretions diminish as we age. See a physician who can conduct stool and digestive analyses to see how well you are digesting your food. There are many nutritional preparations that can greatly assist the digestion of food. When appropriately used, these can prove to be some of the most valuable supplements for senior citizens.

Freshly prepared vegetable juice from tomatoes, carrots, celery, cantaloupe, beets, or any produce can be a valuable food for older adults. It is high in vitamins, minerals, and other valuable substances and is very easily assimilated. Go to a health food store that makes fresh juices and try some. If you like it, buy a high-quality juicer and a book to show you how to get started. It should be part of your daily routine.

No matter what your chronological age, it is never too late to enjoy the benefits of optimal nutrition.

SUMMING UP

Older adults should:
- Take optimal levels of most essential nutrients
- Avoid supplements of iron and vitamin D unless prescribed by a physician
- Consume an abundant supply of antioxidants through food and supplements
- Make sure that they are digesting and absorbing their nutrients well
- Take a standardized ginkgo extract
- Find a physician who will avoid the needless use of prescription medications

CHAPTER 26

Nutritional Strategies for Stopping Smoking

Cigarettes don't kill you—death does.
> —Cigarette company spokesperson

C IGARETTES DESTROY THE HEALTH OF more people throughout the world than any other factor. They cost America $50 billion per year and cause over two million preventable deaths annually. Smoking increases the risk of cancer, heart disease, and lung disease. It wrinkles skin, and causes a deterioration of virtually every organ and gland in the body.

Secondhand smoke is almost as deadly. This is especially true for children. Over two hundred research papers from throughout the world document a significant increase in respiratory disease, ear infections, and other health problems in children who breathe passive smoke. In infants, it causes irreversible lung damage.[388]

WHAT IS AN ADAPTOGEN?

An adaptogen normalizes metabolism. It is a tonic that helps the body in whatever area it needs it. Cigarettes are adaptogens. They help the body function better under stress and normalize metabolism in many ways. They stimulate the body when it is tired and calm it down when it is anxious. They are the number one adaptogen in America.

Cigarettes initially help the body deal with stress. In the long run, however, they make it less able to manage it. They destroy important stress-managing nutrients such as vitamin C, vitamin E, beta carotene, vitamin A and essential fatty acids. They also leach calcium from the body. Calcium is necessary for a relaxed, healthy nervous system. By suppressing appetite, cigarettes decrease the amount of stress managing nutrients consumed as well.

THE RIGHT DIET

There are positive ways to help the body deal with stress. The first is to eat enough protein. Protein is needed to detoxify many of the substances in cigarettes. It also supports the adrenal glands, which sit atop each kidney and help the body balance blood sugar and energy levels. Sugar and white flour products must also be avoided. They deplete the body of nutrients, lower energy levels, create food cravings, and decrease the body's ability to handle stress. Alcohol and coffee should also be avoided for the same reasons.

An Adaptogenic Oil

Virgin flaxseed oil may be the most important food for smokers, especially those trying to quit. One to three tablespoons of virgin flaxseed oil on salads or in yogurt can help the body manage stress and will decrease the need for the stress-managing effects of cigarettes. Flaxseed oil helps the body maintain even energy levels, and is one of the most nourishing foods for the nervous system.[389]

Ginseng: The Ultimate Adaptogen

Siberian ginseng, more properly called *Eleutherococcus senticosus*, is the best-studied adaptogenic herb. If blood sugar or pressure is high or low, or the immune system is underfunctioning or overstimulated, ginseng will help normalize these functions. Ginseng also nourishes the adrenal glands and helps the body deal with stress more effectively. As cigarette smoking, stress, poor eating habits, alcohol, and overwork stress the body, adaptogenic herbs like Eleutherococcus play an invaluable role promoting health and helping one to quit. It also helps the body cleanse itself of the many toxins in cigarettes. Other valuable tonic herbs include licorice root, saw palmetto, schizandra, and gotu kola.

Oatstraw

An herb that is an excellent tonic for the nervous system, oatstraw is very helpful during the detoxification process and can give the body the strength to break addictions.

These nutritional suggestions will not make you quit—you have to have the desire and the persistence to begin with. For many people, it takes repeated attempts. Yet these nutrients are essential to the quitting process. They strengthen and detoxify the body and replace the valuable adaptogenic properties of cigarettes, which many still desire long after their addiction to nicotine has been broken.

Summing Up

The following daily regimen of nutrients is invaluable to the quitting process:

Siberian ginseng	2–8 capsules (standardized extract)
(*Eleutherococcus senticosus*)	
Virgin flax oil	1–3 tablespoons
Oatstraw tincture	1–3 droppers in 8 ounces of water
B complex	50 mg
Vitamin C	1–10 grams
Vitamin E	400 IUs
Calcium	500 mg
Magnesium	400 mg
Zinc picolinate	25–75 mg

All smokers should take a full complement of antioxidants, especially vitamin A and beta-carotene. If you have high blood pressure, begin with no more than 100 IUs of vitamin E and do so under a doctor's supervision.

Why are the people in cigarette ads never smoking? Do tobacco companies not want the young, fun, and attractive image they portray in their ads associated with something as negative as cigarettes?

CHAPTER 27

Top Ten Ways to Enhance Your Lovemaking Ability

1. *Eat a Healthy Diet.* A balanced diet rich in all beneficial nutrients is essential for a healthy sex life. Hydrogenated or refined oils, sugar, refined flours, and fried foods clog arteries and upset the balance of hormones needed for overall wellness and sexual health.

2. *Exercise.* Aerobic exercise such as walking, jogging, or swimming is a very important way to keep all body systems functioning well. Aerobic exercise enhances circulation, stamina, and heart health, and promotes the overall well-being needed for an energetic love life.

3. *Manage Stress.* Stress, whether emotional, financial, or job-related, can make it difficult for the brain and nervous system to enjoy or even allow the act of lovemaking. Relaxation techniques such as moderate exercise, music, epsom salt baths, and meditation can help keep stress from interfering with your sex life.

4. *Enhance Intestinal Health.* Candida overgrowth, parasites, or a proliferation of bad bacteria in the GI tract can upset the health of the body and decrease libido. Beneficial bacteria such as acidophilus and bifidobacterium can help relieve these problems. Any intestinal problem requires the guidance of a knowledgeable nutritionist.

5. *Avoid Alcohol.* Alcohol is a sedative, and will diminish sexual performance and the pleasure derived from it. Alcohol also depletes nutrients such as magnesium, zinc, and B vitamins, all of which are needed for a healthy sex life.

6. *Take Specific Nutrients:* **Minerals** of all kinds are needed for healthy sexual function. One of the most important is **zinc**, which many people are deficient in. Zinc is critical for the health of the prostate and for testosterone production in men. Zinc is also needed for female hormone balance.

Potassium is a very important mineral for muscle tone and high energy levels. Vegetables and fresh vegetable juices are high in potassium, as are nuts, seeds, and most unrefined whole foods.

7. Essential fats found in flaxseed oil and GLA supplements can enhance sexual function. They also feed the nervous system, which must be optimally nourished on a daily basis for a healthy sex life to exist.

8. Herbal products of many kinds have been used for centuries as aphrodisiacs, and science is just beginning to document their effectiveness. Siberian ginseng as well as other members of the ginseng family can increase sex drive and endurance. Saw palmetto is an excellent tonic for male reproductive health, with particular benefit for the prostate gland. Damiana, dong quai, and licorice have long been celebrated as female tonics. Ginkgo enhances circulation in the brain, the most important sex organ in the body. Ginkgo also stimulates circulation to other areas as well. Encapsulated standardized extracts are recommended when using ginseng, ginkgo, or saw palmetto. They deliver the most reliable results.

9. Dimethylglycine or DMG is a nonvitamin nutrient that increases stamina and tissue oxygen levels. Many have found that it increases lovemaking endurance and enjoyment.

10. L-Arginine is an amino acid that is useful for men who have trouble maintaining an erection. L-Arginine, like all amino acids, should be taken on an empty stomach for maximum benefit. Four grams of L-Arginine per day has also been found to increase sperm count in 80% of men with low counts. Avoid L-Arginine if you have herpes.

PART IV
Health Problems and Nutrition

CHAPTER 28

What Is Hypoglycemia?

HYPOGLYCEMIA OR LOW BLOOD SUGAR refers to the body's inability to maintain normal levels of sugar in the blood. Sugar is the main source of fuel for the body, and sugar levels must remain steady. Otherwise, the brain and other organs cannot function normally. When sugar levels become undesirably low, as can occur between meals or soon after sweets are eaten, the following problems can occur:

- Food cravings, especially for sugar and starchy foods
- Depression
- Fatigue
- Headaches
- Anger
- PMS
- Dizziness
- Fainting
- Arrhythmias
- Inability to concentrate
- Panic attacks

Most of us at one time or another experience a degree of low blood sugar. If we are tired or moody because we have not eaten for many hours, it is a sign that our blood sugar is low. Yet chronic hypoglycemia is more than mere moodiness associated with a lack of food. It is a sign that the organs that help balance blood sugar, such as the adrenal glands and the pancreas, aren't doing a good enough job. Fortunately, the symptoms of hypoglycemia can be eliminated with a diet of whole foods, frequent meals, and carefully chosen nutritional supplements.

The Glucose Tolerance Test

How do you know if you have hypoglycemia? One way is to have a physician administer a four hour glucose tolerance test. In this test, you arrive at the physician's office in the morning without having eaten anything. You then drink a solution of sugar that assaults your body with more sugar than you are likely to consume in a day. Your blood is then taken every hour for at least four hours and the sugar levels are recorded. If your blood sugar goes too high or too low or there are steep dives between readings, your body is showing it cannot control blood sugar well.

Your symptoms during the glucose tolerance test are just as important as your blood readings. If you are fainting, have a headache, or feel dizzy or nauseous during the test, you can be sure you have hypoglycemia no matter what the blood readings are. Many physicians pronounce a patient free of low blood sugar based on the blood sugar readings even though the patient has fallen asleep or fainted. Are they treating a person or a test?

An easier way to determine whether you have blood sugar instability is to examine your symptoms. This may not be as definitive as a glucose tolerance test, but many do not have access to a physician who administers such tests. Since the treatment for hypoglycemia is a healthy diet and lifestyle, which often effectively removes the symptoms, many have found this an effective way of assessing and treating their blood sugar instability.

The following are signs of low blood sugar:

- I get headaches or feel weak, shaky, or like fainting if I haven't eaten for three or more hours.
- I often crave sugar.
- My energy levels are more stable when I eat meals higher in protein.
- Sometimes I notice that I get angry when I haven't eaten for more than three hours.
- I get very moody or tired when I eat sugar.
- I feel best when I eat small meals throughout the day.

Saying yes to any of these questions does not classify you as a hypoglycemic. Agreement to most or all of them, however, is a sign that you need to change your diet to one that is more effective at balancing blood sugar.

Low blood sugar comes in varying degrees of severity. Many who can pass a glucose tolerance test are often told, "You do not have low blood sugar." Yet they may have mild blood sugar problems that only come up after many hours without eating or when they are under stress. They need to change their diet as well. They cannot expect their energy levels to remain constant without eating small meals that contain protein at regular intervals throughout the day.

Adrenal Burnout and Hypoglycemia

One of the causes of hypoglycemia is tired adrenal glands. The adrenal glands sit on top of each kidney and are very important for keeping blood sugar balanced. When we are stressed over prolonged periods of time, or use sugar, coffee, or allergenic foods on a regular basis, we burn out our adrenal glands and set the stage for low blood sugar. That is why helping the adrenal glands with vitamin C, protein, rest, and ginseng extracts has been found helpful in restoring blood sugar balance. It helps repair the body's own blood sugar balancing mechanisms.

THE DIET FOR HYPOGLYCEMIA

Following simple dietary principles will relieve the symptoms of hypoglycemia:

- Remove all sugar and concentrated sweeteners, refined flours, and processed foods from the diet.
- Make sure you are eating adequate amounts of protein throughout the day.
- Consume moderate amounts of healthy fats from raw nuts, virgin flax oil, olives, and avocados.
- Consume whole, unrefined foods low on the glycemic index and high in fiber.
- Avoid alcohol.
- Avoid fruit juice.
- Take dietary supplements that have proven to be helpful such as chromium, zinc, licorice, and ginseng.

No sugar or concentrated sweeteners in any form. Sugar will not only lead to unstable blood sugar but will further exhaust the blood sugar balancing mechanisms in the body. Barley malt, maple syrup, succanat, honey, and all so-called "natural" sweeteners should be eliminated.

Eat protein. This is the single most important nutrient for hypoglycemics. Three to four ounces with both lunch and dinner is recommended. Eating all your protein at one meal is not acceptable. Protein must be distributed between at least two meals to help balance blood sugar.

Protein is like oxygen: You can't store it in your body, and you need a constant supply of it throughout the day. Have you ever heard anyone say, "I can't breathe now, I'm too busy. I'll breathe tonight?" Of course not. This approach does not work for protein, either. If you go all day without eating protein, your body will not be able to balance blood sugar and energy levels.

Many people, especially women, eat a bagel with coffee for breakfast, a green salad for lunch, and pasta or some other carbohydrate food for dinner. Their bodies are literally suffocating on such low protein regimes, sending their blood sugar and food cravings out of control.

Protein has many benefits:

- Protein supports the adrenal glands, the pancreas, and the liver, all of which need to be adequately nourished in order to keep blood sugar balanced.
- Roughly half of the amino acids that make up protein can be turned into sugar by the liver and keep energy levels steady.
- Inadequate protein consumption leads to cravings for carbohydrate foods, such as sugar and bread, that perpetuate the unstable blood sugar cycle.

Don't be afraid of all foods that contain fat. The right fats play a key role in balancing blood sugar and reducing cravings and mood swings.

- Fat increases satiety.
- Fat enhances the flavor of food.
- Fat slows the digestion of food, allowing it to be released into the bloodstream more slowly for more constant energy levels.
- Beneficial fats such as flax oil enhance energy and mood levels.
- Almonds, walnuts, olives, and avocados all balance blood sugar.

The Glycemic Index

All carbohydrate containing foods—potatoes, lentils, pasta, carrots, fruits, or candy—are eventually broken down into sugar and enter the bloodstream. Yet the rate at which they do so differs for each food. The rate at which the sugars or carbohydrates in a food enter the bloodstream is known as a food's "glycemic index." The discovery of the differing glycemic indexes was groundbreaking. It demonstrated that all carbohydrates are not created equal. Each one has a different effect on blood sugar levels and is digested and enters the bloodstream at a different speed. The higher the value, the more quickly it enters the bloodstream. Lower is better. It means the food is more gradually released and digested and is less likely to cause blood sugar fluctuations and stress the body.

GLYCEMIC INDEX FOR COMMON FOODS

Fructose	20	Corn flakes	80	Apples	39
Glucose	100	Puffed rice	95	Beans	31
Honey	75	Bananas	62	Lentils	29
Maltose	105	Beets	64	Nuts	13
Sucrose	60	Carrots, cooked	36	Oranges	40
Bread, white	69	Corn	59	Raisins	64
Bread, whole grain	72	Peas	39	Milk	34
Pasta	45	Potatoes, baked	98	Juice, orange	46
Rice, brown	66	Potatoes, new, boiled	70	Ice cream	36[390]
Cereal, bran	51	Sweet potatoes	48		
Cereal, wheat	67	Sausages	28		

Should hypoglycemics and diabetics eat everything with low numbers and avoid everything with high ones? Not really. While glycemic index is an important tool to help us understand which foods can turn into blood sugar more quickly, it does not tell us everything about a food's effect on our metabolism. While raw nuts are health-promoting, aged meats like sausage are not. While fructose has a very low number, it is still a concentrated sweet that should only be consumed when in fruit. Many foods are combined to make a meal. The high glycemic index of foods like potatoes can be blunted if eaten with flax oil or butter, which will slow its digestion.

The glycemic index demonstrates that foods like lentils, nuts, and beans are excellent foods for hypoglycemics. Because these foods turn into sugar more slowly, they help provide balanced energy over longer periods of time. This is critical for removing the symptoms of hypoglycemia.

Fiber. Fiber is the unabsorbed portion of food that helps the digestive process and usually slows the release of carbohydrates in food. The value of whole, unrefined grain products is not just that they are higher in vitamins, minerals, and essential fatty acids. Their fiber content helps the body digest the carbohydrates in food more slowly. High-fiber foods are excellent at helping balance blood sugar and energy levels.

IMPORTANT NUTRIENTS FOR HYPOGLYCEMICS

Our adrenal glands need generous amounts of vitamin C and B complex to function optimally. Pantothenic acid and vitamin A are also of particular importance. Other nutrients that help to balance blood sugar include magnesium, zinc, chromium, glutamine, and ginseng.

Magnesium

Magnesium is a very important nutrient for balancing blood sugar. Those better nourished with magnesium balance blood sugar more effectively. Magnesium affects both insulin secretion and its action. This may account for its beneficial effect on blood sugar balance.[391]

Zinc

Zinc is another key nutrient for hypoglycemics. It is very helpful in controlling sugar cravings. Between 25 and 50 milligrams of zinc picolinate per day is recommended for hypoglycemics. It should be balanced with copper if taken over long periods of time. Stress increases zinc requirements.

Chromium

Chromium is an essential supplement for hypoglycemics. Chromium helps to balance blood sugar and the hormone insulin, both of which must be kept under control if energy and mood levels are to remain even. Hypoglycemics rarely have enough chromium. Between 200 and 600 micrograms of chromium picolinate per day is highly recommended.

Glutamine

Glutamine is an amino acid that can energize the body and eliminate sugar cravings. It is also a very important nutrient for the health of the GI tract. Many hypoglycemics find that 500 to 1,000 milligrams of L-Glutamine taken on an empty stomach with water is a great way to get energy that they used to derive from dosing up on sugar and coffee.

Ginseng

Ginseng (*Eleutherococcus senticosus*) standardized extracts have been found very helpful at strengthening the adrenal glands and increasing their ability to balance blood sugar. Ginseng standardized extracts are the most important herbal products for those with low blood sugar.

AVOID STIMULANTS

Coffee, chocolate, caffeine-containing over-the-counter medications, ephedra, kola nut, and anything that acts as a stimulant on the adrenal system will only further tire out the blood-sugar-balancing mechanisms of the body. Avoid them. Although they may give you temporary energy, in the long run they will only make you more tired and make your blood sugar more unstable.

HERBS TO AVOID

Raw garlic and garlic powder, pau d'arco, goldenseal, and cayenne or hot pepper are botanicals with many benefits. However, all of these also have blood-sugar-lowering effects and may not be ideal for persons with hypoglycemia. These natural products can create fatigue and depression in hypoglycemics. Hot spices of all kinds should be used in small amounts by those with low blood sugar. Each hypoglycemic will find different levels of these substances that they may be able to tolerate.

EXERCISE

Moderate amounts of exercise are essential for hypoglycemics. Twenty minutes of walking, jogging, or some other aerobic exercise three times a week will significantly improve insulin metabolism. When the cells of the body respond to insulin better, sugar cravings decrease and energy and mood levels even out.

SUMMING UP

Hypoglycemia is a decreased ability to balance blood sugar. It occurs in different people in different degrees. The treatment for hypoglycemia is a healthy diet rich in essential nutrients.

The following guidelines can help keep blood sugar levels stable:

- Avoid sugar and all concentrated sweeteners
- Consume adequate protein, at least two 3–4 ounce servings per day
- Consume foods high in fiber, low in glycemic index
- Augment a healthy diet with magnesium, zinc, chromium, standardized ginseng extract, and other helpful supplements.

Usually, once these lifestyle habits are adopted, the fatigue, dizziness, mood swings, PMS, and other problems associated with hypoglycemia become a thing of the past. The most difficult thing for hypoglycemics to do is to break old patterns and understand that faddish ultra-low-fat, high-carbohydrate diets are not right for them.

CHAPTER 29

Lowering Blood Pressure Naturally

No illness which can be treated by diet should be treated by any other means.

—Maimonides

HIGH BLOOD PRESSURE PATIENTS ARE often told that they must stay on their medication for life. That's like telling you once your car burns oil, it always will and you should buy more oil every week. There is a conflict of interest. The late Dr. Robert Mendelssohn said every good physician should be in the business of putting himself out of business by teaching his or her patients how to stay healthy. That should especially be the case with hypertension. While some people may actually require medication to keep their blood pressure under control, most can lower it through losing weight, consuming optimal levels of blood-pressure-lowering nutrients, and stress management.

The scarceness of physicians who know how to manipulate blood pressure through natural means often creates the need for nutritional self-care. Foods and supplements that lower blood pressure are quite safe, but don't neglect to have your blood pressure checked regularly by a qualified health professional. You cannot let high blood pressure persist, and it may take time for natural therapies to work. Physician supervision is always recommended. You may need medication until you know how nutrition and lifestyle changes affect your blood pressure.

High blood pressure is unknown in primitive cultures that eat a diet of unprocessed foods. Hypertension is another ailment that we bring upon ourselves with refined grains, sugar, refined oils, margarine, overeating, inactivity, stress, and smoking.

If you are overweight, begin a program of gradual weight loss. Even beginning to lose weight will lower blood pressure. Keeping weight off is one of the most important strategies for controlling blood pressure. Even losing a pound a week is a significant stride in the right direction. In fact, for hypertensives, slow weight loss of one to two pounds a week is ideal. Anything faster may deplete important blood-pressure-regulating minerals such as magnesium and potassium.

High blood pressure is often accompanied by high blood levels of insulin. High insulin levels may cause high blood pressure. High levels of insulin will also make weight loss more difficult. A diet high in carbohydrates may not be ideal for hypertensives, for it will perpetuate high insulin levels. It will also worsen food cravings. Hypertensives who are overweight should restrict carbohydrates—grains, beans, legumes, and fruits—to no more than 40% of their diet in an effort to get their insulin levels back to normal.

Foods that must be eliminated from the diet of hypertensives:

- Salty foods or processed foods high in sodium
- Caffeinated coffee
- Caffeinated tea
- Alcohol
- Sugar
- Margarine and fried foods
- Refined white flours and supermarket oils
- Stimulants such as ephedra (ma huang) and kola nut

Regular aerobic exercise such as walking can help lower blood pressure. It should be done only with your physician's approval.

Nutritional Factors that Affect Blood Pressure

Sugar
All refined sweeteners are particularly damaging to hypertensives. Sugar stresses the glands and organs that control blood pressure. Sugar also depletes many valuable nutrients needed to lower blood pressure. Sugar also raises insulin levels, which in turn may raise blood pressure.

Garlic
Garlic has been shown in many studies to lower blood pressure. Both fresh garlic and garlic supplements are effective. Onions are also helpful.[392]

Celery

Studies at the University of Chicago have shown that celery lowers blood pressure by relaxing smooth muscles that line the blood vessel walls. The amount needed to lower blood pressure is four celery stalks per day.

Fish Oils

Fish oils are well documented for their ability to reduce blood pressure at a dose of 2 grams of EPA per day.[393] However, if blood pressure is uncontrolled or unknown, fish oils are not recommended. They should only be taken when blood pressure is under control.[394] Fish oils alone may not lower blood pressure sufficiently for some hypertensives. Minerals such as calcium, magnesium, and potassium, and foods such as garlic and onions should be combined with EPA for an overall nutritional approach to hypertension.[395]

Vitamin C

Vitamin C is lower in those with higher diastolic blood pressure.[396] A study of sixty-nine adults found that vitamin C levels were inversely related to blood pressure. Those with the most vitamin C in their blood had the lowest blood pressure. One gram per day decreased blood pressure significantly.[397]

Calcium and Magnesium

These two minerals are essential for anyone with hypertension. There are a myriad of studies that demonstrate that they both lower blood pressure naturally.[398, 399, 400] Calcium and magnesium have also been used to treat the toxemia of pregnancy. Supplements of 1,000 milligrams of calcium with 400–600 milligrams of magnesium per day are the amounts most find helpful.

Potassium

This mineral also keeps blood pressure in normal ranges. Low levels raise blood pressure and lead to an increase in the excretion of calcium. Potassium depletion also causes the body to retain more sodium, which can also increase blood pressure.[401]

Potassium supplementation lowers blood pressure.[402] The longer potassium supplements are taken, the more effective potassium's blood-pressure-lowering effects will be.[403] Potassium supplements should always be combined with magnesium. Magnesium deficiency makes it difficult for the body to hold on to potassium. Forty percent of those who are low in potassium have also been found to be low in magnesium, proving the maxim that nutritional deficiencies are usually multiple.[404]

Increase the potassium in your diet by consuming more whole, unprocessed fruits, vegetables, grains, beans, and legumes. Eat fresh meat products and avoid processed or canned varieties. Freshly prepared vegetable juices are an extraordinary source of potassium. They are also rich in magnesium, vitamin C, and other nutrients that benefit hypertensives.

Chromium Picolinate
Chromium picolinate is helpful for hypertensives for many reasons. It has been shown to:
- Control sugar cravings
- Lower insulin levels
- Increase weight loss
- Increase lean tissue growth

All of these are important for lowering blood pressure and losing weight. Between 200 and 600 micrograms per day is the amount most find helpful.

Taurine
Taurine is an amino acid that lowers blood pressure remarkably well. Taurine is made by the body in small amounts, but for people with high blood pressure, supplementation is required. The effective dose is 1–3 grams per day with meals in divided amounts.[405] Taurine has been shown to help insulin be more effectively taken up by body cells. This may be a mechanism by which it may help lower blood pressure.[406]

CoEnzyme Q10
CoQ10 is a non-vitamin nutrient that is often deficient in hypertensives. It lowers blood pressure when taken as a supplement. Typical doses for lowering pressure range between 50 and 75 milligrams per day. CoEnzyme Q10 also protects against damage to the body that is caused by hypertension.[407] Coenzyme Q10 also helps promote weight loss which in turn will reduce blood pressure.[408]

EAT LESS SALT

Sodium is overconsumed by Americans, and there are good reasons to eat less. Most of the sodium Americans eat does not come from the salt shaker. It only accounts for 15% of the salt in the American diet. Processed foods are the major source. Sodium can lead to imbalances in many minerals and causes calcium depletion. It also increases the risk for hardening of the arteries.

Sodium promotes stomach cancer. A Japanese study demonstrated a nearly complete correlation between urinary salt excretion and stomach cancer mortality. A 40% reduction in salt intake could result in as much as a 65% reduction in stomach cancer rates.[409] A Turkish study further confirmed this hypothesis, showing that those with stomach cancer had a higher consumption of salt and salted foods than healthy subjects.[410]

Salt restriction has only been shown to have a modest blood-pressure-lowering effect in a percentage of the population called "salt-sensitive." About half of hypertensives appear to be salt-sensitive. Obesity is a far more significant cause of hypertension in the United States. Eat less salt—just do not go to extremes and remove all food sources of sodium from your diet.[411, 412]

The easiest way to eat the right amount of sodium is to consume foods as unprocessed and as close to their natural state as possible. Avoid all processed foods. Do not use the salt shaker. Ideally, salt and sodium intake should be kept under 1,000 milligrams or 1 gram per day, very easily achieved on a diet of natural foods.

Cadmium

Cadmium is a toxic metal in cigarette paper that is often found in high amounts in hypertensives. Cadmium raises blood pressure. It is also associated with more aggressive behavior that may also raise blood pressure and deplete blood-pressure-lowering minerals. A hair analysis can show whether cadmium levels are dangerously high.

Summing Up

- Maintain your weight at an ideal level.
- If you are overweight, lose weight gradually and permanently.
- If you are using diuretic medications, work with your physician and a nutritionist to see if a combination of

weight loss, optimal nutrition, and moderate exercise can
reduce or eliminate your need for these life-shortening
medications.

- Take optimal amounts of all blood-pressure-lowering nu-
  trients such as calcium, magnesium and taurine.
- Eat garlic and onions liberally.
- Exercise on a regular basis. Walking may be the ideal
  exercise for hypertensives.
- Don't smoke, and avoid alcohol.
- Drink as much fresh vegetable juice as possible.
- Use stress-reducing techniques such as yoga, meditation,
  biofeedback, and laughter.

CHAPTER 30

Does Cholesterol Cause Heart Disease?

*Understanding of our most serious health disorder, athero-
genetic disease, is now confused, its management at a stale-
mate. The proposal that obstructive vascular disease is caused
by hypercholesterolemia resulting from an excess of saturated fat and cholesterol in the diet has been repeatedly
tested and found to be wrong.*
— George V. Mann, M.D., *Lancet*, May 21, 1994

YOU TURN ON THE TELEVISION and see the governor holding a news conference. He is announcing that electricity will be banned immediately. The recent death of three children due to a downed electrical wire has outraged everyone. "Enough is enough," he says. "For complete safety, we have no other choice." Then, due to the loss of power, your set goes off.

Wait a second, you say—I like electricity. I use it correctly, and it doesn't cause any problems. This is ridiculous!

That is precisely what researchers say in response to those who blame cholesterol for causing heart disease. Cholesterol is entirely beneficial until a lack of insulating nutrients causes it to be mishandled by the body. Not only is cholesterol harmless when consumed as part of a healthy diet, it is beneficial.

Cholesterol is a high-molecular-weight alcohol known as a sterol. It is found in every cell in the body. Without it, the body could not make hormones, vitamin D, and the membranes of our cells. Cholesterol is so vital that if you eat none, your body will manufacture it.

THE GREAT NUTRIENT-DEPLETING EXPERIMENT

We like to believe that in all areas of human endeavor, things are constantly improving. However, the quality of food eaten in civilized countries took a turn for the worse in the twentieth century. The great nutrient-deprivation experiment occurred. In this century, as never before, our health has been devastated by removing essential nutrients from our food supply, adding back potentially harmful ones like vitamin D and iron, creating new toxic foods like hydrogenated shortenings and margarines, and eating too many refined polyunsaturated vegetable oils. The dramatic increase in sugar consumption that also occurred in this century has also been detrimental. An epidemic of degenerative diseases has resulted.

It is no surprise that the epidemic of coronary artery disease began a few years after this nutrient-deprivation experiment began. Coronary artery disease, which will hereafter be referred to as heart disease, is largely a twentieth-century phenomenon. It appeared in the medical literature for the first time in 1912 in the *Journal of the American Medical Association.* Even in the teens, the degeneration of arteries was so rare that the famous cardiologist Dr. Paul Dudley White spent ten years looking for it and found only three cases.[413] Today over sixty million Americans have some degree of coronary disease. One in three persons will die from it. The imbalance in nutrients that occurs due to our modern deprivation experiment upsets the ability of the body to handle cholesterol correctly.

CHOLESTEROL OXIDATION

Cholesterol is an innocent and essential substance that is always traveling down the highway of your bloodstream. Then, out of nowhere, a drunk driver known as a free radical slams into it. Careening out of control, cholesterol slams into your artery wall. The body then covers up the whole accident scene with plaque. If the artery is not strengthened where it had been weakened by the accident, it might rupture. Result? Your arteries are thinner. When a clot from platelets that are too sticky comes down the highway, it gets stuck where the road is too narrow. Depending on which artery gets blocked, you will either have a heart attack, stroke, or a dangerous cutoff of circulation somewhere else in your body.

The whole thing begins with free radicals. Cholesterol is merely part of the process because it is ubiquitous. Free radicals cannot do their damage as long as we get enough of the antioxidants that neutralize them. If cholesterol doesn't oxidize, it is harmless.

WHERE DO FREE RADICALS COME FROM?

Free radicals are unstable compounds that come from smog and stress, and are natural byproducts of the everyday metabolism of our bodies. When we are optimally nourished we can control them with a series of nutrients and enzymes known as antioxidants.

The antioxidant protection system fails only under two circumstances:

- When we do not get enough of the protective antioxidant nutrients such as vitamins C, E, beta-carotene, zinc, selenium, and CoQ10, and fail to eat enough produce, protein, and acidophilus-rich dairy products.
- When free radicals outnumber our defense system. This can happen when we smoke, drink excessively, undergo constant stress, have excess iron, overeat, lose weight, breathe polluted air, get too much sun, get too little sleep, have bad bacteria in our intestinal tract, or eat fried foods, margarine, or too many refined polyunsaturated vegetable oils.

Free radicals not only oxidize cholesterol and start the process that thins arteries. They also damage the calcium pump that controls the amount of calcium in your heart cells. If the pump is damaged, calcium cannot be pumped out of heart cells. Too much calcium in heart cells will stop the heart from beating. Inflammation in and around the heart also plays a pivotal role in heart disease. Inflammation increases the amount of free radicals in the heart, and these free radicals damage the ability of the heart to break down food and keep itself beating. So free radicals from inflammation keep the heart from beating, and in so doing, shorten the life of the heart in another way. And free radicals make platelets more sticky, increasing the likelihood that they will create unwanted clots that can lead to a heart attack or a stroke.

DOES MODERN MEDICINE HAVE THE ANSWER?

Modern medicine would have you believe that deaths from heart and artery disease are declining, but this is not true. According to statistics from the American Heart Association and the National Center for Health Statistics, only 490,000 heart and vessel deaths occurred in 1989.[414] Yet the same statistics given out by these organizations shows 945,000 deaths were attributed to "major cardiovascular diseases" in that same year. As Brian Leibovitz, Ph.D., points out,

> Apparently, 455,000 people died in 1989 from "heart and vessel diseases" that were not "cardiovascular diseases." It would be of more than passing interest to learn what mystery diseases of the heart and vessels—but unrelated to the cardiovascular system—killed almost half a million people in 1989.[415]

The rates for heart disease in America are not declining. Medications, bypass surgery, and other medical interventions cost billions of dollars per year and have not been shown to reduce the fatalities from heart disease. Perhaps deceptive manipulation of numbers is needed to prevent public outcry against the current unproven medical techniques that are used to combat heart disease. The $43 billion spent annually on these ineffective remedies is arguably the biggest waste of money in American history.

PREVENTING HEART DISEASE WITH OPTIMAL NUTRITION

The evidence is mounting that the real solution to heart disease is eliminating all refined, processed foods, limiting the sources of free radicals in our diet and lifestyle, and increasing the amounts of antioxidant nutrients we consume.

The B Complex

If you fail to consume optimal amounts of B complex vitamins, an artery-damaging amino acid known as homocysteine can form in your blood.[416] According to a study in the *New England Journal of Medicine*, 42% of the patients with cerebrovascular disease and 30% of those with cardiovascular disease have elevated homocysteine levels.[417] Patients with even slightly elevated levels of homocysteine have over three times the risk of a heart attack.[418, 419] Unless B vitamin nutrition is optimal— beyond the RDA—homocysteine levels will elevate in susceptible persons. Fifty milligrams of B complex per day will give the body everything it needs to metabolize homocysteine into harmless byproducts.[420]

Vitamin B₆

Vitamin B_6 in particular has many mechanisms by which it prevents heart disease. It prevents cholesterol from a damaging process known as glycosylation, which in turn clogs arteries. B_6 keeps platelets from dangerously aggregating. B_6 is necessary for normal collagen metabolism and for maintaining the integrity of the vascular wall. Animal studies show that a B_6-deficient diet will lead to clogged arteries.[421]

Beta-Carotene

Beta-carotene is the orange-yellow pigment found in fruits and vegetables. It plays a very important role in the prevention of heart and artery disease. It is found in significant amounts in carrots, sweet potatoes, yellow and orange peppers, apricots, and leafy green vegetables. Supplements are recommended for those who do not consume five or more servings of fruits and vegetables per day. According to the USDA, 90% of us don't eat enough produce. Recommended amounts: 25,000 to 200,000 IUs per day. Beta-carotene is a fat-soluble nutrient and should be taken with a meal that contains some fat. Ultra-low-fat diets may not allow for adequate beta-carotene absorption.[422]

Beta-carotene inhibits the laying down of plaque in artery walls. Beta-carotene also concentrates in plaques that have already developed and stops their further progression. In addition, beta-carotene increases levels of HDL cholesterol, the more protective form of cholesterol.[423, 424, 425] A study of 333 patients who took 50 milligrams of beta-carotene showed that such supplementation reduced major cardiovascular events by 50%.[426] Lycopene is a carotenoid found in tomatoes that plays an important role along with beta-carotene in protecting LDL cholesterol from sticking to artery walls.[427]

Vitamin C

Vitamin C plays such a valuable role in preventing heart disease that Linus Pauling described heart disease as an early stage of scurvy. While vitamin E and beta-carotene can slow the oxidation of cholesterol once it has begun, only vitamin C can completely prevent it from occurring. Persons with higher intakes of vitamin C have also been found to have a higher level of beneficial HDL cholesterol.[428, 429] Less cholesterol is absorbed from foods when vitamin C is present.[430] Vitamin C has repeatedly been found to be at lower levels in those who develop cardiovascular disease.[431, 432, 433] Low levels of vitamin C are considered by many researchers to be a risk factor for heart disease.[434, 435, 436]

Vitamin C is found in fruits, vegetables, and potatoes. Few of us could eat the amount of produce necessary to consume optimal levels of this nutrient. Recommended amounts: 500 milligrams or more per day. Vitamin C should be taken in divided doses throughout the day for maximum protection.

Vitamin E

A recent study conducted by the World Health Organization concluded that inadequate vitamin E consumption is the single biggest risk factor for heart disease. Vitamin E is another powerful preventer of cholesterol oxidation. Vitamin E and vitamin A levels together could be used to successfully predict 73% of the ischemic heart disease mortality in one study of Europeans aged forty to forty-nine.[437] Not only does vitamin E keep cholesterol from sticking to artery walls, but it also lowers cholesterol levels as well.[438]

No foods contain significant amounts of vitamin E. The only way to increase body levels of vitamin E is to take a supplement. One hundred IUs is the minimum beneficial dose. More optimal doses range between 400 and 800 IUS per day. Persons with high blood pressure or using blood-thinning medication should consult their physicians before using vitamin E supplements.[439, 440, 441]

Magnesium

Magnesium is the most important mineral for heart health. The heart uses calcium to contract and needs magnesium to relax. The severely magnesium-deficient heart will stop beating, for it cannot relax. Physicians performing heart surgery have actually watched these magnesium-deficient heart attacks occur. They can happen independent of all other factors. Up to 25% of all heart attacks occur in people with clear coronary arteries. They are probably caused by a lack of this crucial mineral.[442] Magnesium is also an antioxidant and can compensate for low levels of vitamin E. Most Americans are deficient and need to supplement with 400 to 600 milligrams. Serum magnesium is useless in assessing magnesium levels. Most physicians never check their heart patients' magnesium levels with reliable, inexpensive tests such as the magnesium loading test.

Trace Minerals

Selenium and chromium are two trace minerals needed in small, regular amounts for heart disease prevention. Modern farming methods have greatly reduced the amount of these minerals in our foods. They are mandatory supplements. The latest research recommends supplementing with at least 100 micrograms of each per day.

Low plasma levels of selenium have been found to be a significant risk factor for heart disease.[443] Many population studies have shown that selenium is a protective nutrient against the development of heart and artery disease.[444, 445] Selenium protects the heart in many ways: It stimulates the production of the antioxidant enzyme glutathione peroxidase, which protects heart tissue from the high flux of oxygen this organ experiences.[446] Selenium restricts the amount of toxic metals that can build up in the body, such as cadmium, mercury, and lead.

Nuts

There are many studies that show nuts are a valuable source of nutrients that help the body metabolize cholesterol effectively. Both walnuts and almonds have been shown to have positive effects, and should be eaten raw and fresh right from the shell for maximum benefit. Nuts should be refrigerated and purchased from organic growers wherever possible.[447]

Fruits and Vegetables

Fresh produce, while a good source of vitamins and some minerals, may be most valuable as a source of a group of nonvitamin antioxidant compounds known as bioflavonoids and polyphenols. These substances powerfully protect against cholesterol oxidation. While it is a good idea to supplement with vitamins such as C, E, and beta-carotene, it is also important to consume five servings per day of fruits and vegetables. It is the only way to ensure that you are getting significant amounts of these protective factors.

Spices

Foods such as capsicum (red or cayenne pepper), garlic, ginger, turmeric, and a wide variety of other spices have been found to lower cholesterol, nourish the heart, thin the blood, and prevent cholesterol oxidation. Avoid salt and black pepper. Make sure your spices are nonirradiated. All spices contain valuable antioxidant flavonoids. Most spices contain valuable trace minerals as well.

Sunlight

Sunlight is not only the best way to get your vitamin D. Sunshine lowers cholesterol as well. Some patients have seen dramatic lowering of cholesterol levels—as much as one hundred points—after only four days of sunlight treatment. Two hours of sunlight treatment caused a 13% drop in cholesterol in a group of patients with atherosclerosis. Animal studies have shown that sunlight offers complete protection against artery-clogging diets. Human studies have confirmed these effects. Multiple short exposures to sun have been found to be more health-promoting and heart-protecting than single long exposures.[448, 449, 450, 451, 452, 453, 454, 455]

Avoid Excess Iron

High levels of iron in the body can promote free radicals that will in turn oxidize cholesterol. A serum ferritin test will show whether iron is within normal ranges. Avoiding iron-containing supplements and iron-fortified foods is a strategy that helps men and postmenopausal women keep iron levels optimal. *Iron and Your Heart,* by Randall Lauffer, M.D., is a complete and easy-to-read discussion of the many problems excessive iron causes.

Avoid Excess Vitamin D

There is concern that excessive vitamin D from fortified dairy and cereal products, combined with the widespread magnesium deficiency in America, may increase the rate at which plaque is laid down in arteries. Dairy products are fortified with vitamin D to prevent rickets, a form of bone deterioration now rare in civilized countries. It is time to stop fortifying foods with vitamin D. One large serving of fortified cereal with milk packs too high a dose of this hormonelike vitamin.[456]

Xanthine Oxidase

Xanthine oxidase is an enzyme in cow's milk that may cause significant damage to arteries. The process of homogenizing milk allows this enzyme to be absorbed and damage the heart and arteries. New evidence from animal studies demonstrates xanthine oxidase can be absorbed from homogenized milk. Homogenizing milk does more harm than good. Commercial skim milk is free of xanthine oxidase.[457]

Avoid Sugar

Sugar raises cholesterol, triglycerides, and insulin, and increases the stickiness of platelets. Elevated triglyceride levels increase the risk of heart disease. High insulin levels make cholesterol more likely to stick to artery walls. Sugar depletes chromium and increases the cholesterol-raising properties of saturated fats. Sugar consumption will decrease the population of beneficial bacteria that keep cholesterol low. Sugar also interferes with the antioxidant activity of vitamin C, increasing the likelihood that free radicals will damage cholesterol. British nutritionist John Yudkin, Ph.D., has demonstrated the connection between sugar and increased levels of heart disease in his lifelong research and his book *Sweet and Dangerous*.

ARE ROOT CANALS A FACTOR?

Weston Price, D.D.S., conducted research in the early part of this century that questions the safety of root canal procedures. He found that bacteria and toxins can escape from the site of the root canal and infect distant areas of the body. Immune system problems, arthritis, and heart disease all increased in those who had root canals. Further study in this area is needed.

THE ONLY FORM OF CHOLESTEROL TO AVOID: OXIDIZED CHOLESTEROL

Eggs are rich in essential nutrients and are a beneficial, health enhancing food. Countless studies show eggs do not increase the risk for heart disease. Forty-five percent of the fat in eggs is oleic, the kind of fatty acid that is believed to give almonds and olive oil their cholesterol-lowering ability. Eggs have also been shown to raise beneficial HDL cholesterol by 10%.[458]

Powdered, dried eggs found in cake mixes and other processed foods, however, are not beneficial and should be avoided. The same goes for dehydrated milk products and aged meats and cheeses. These foods contain cholesterol that is oxidized and will be much more likely to clog arteries. Fresh meats, poultry, fish, and eggs do not have oxidized cholesterol. Ground hamburger should be used quickly, as grinding exposes the meat to air and increases the rate at which it begins to oxidize.

Unoxidized Cholesterol Does Not Cause Heart Disease

If cholesterol went on trial for causing heart disease, the case would be thrown out for lack of evidence.

- The percentage of the fat in our diet that came from animal products was higher in the pre-heart-disease era.
- Cholesterol consumption has remained the same over the past one hundred years, while heart disease rates have increased almost ten-fold.
- Half of those with heart disease have cholesterol levels that are either normal or low.
- Many primitive groups have no incidence of heart disease even though they have a cholesterol consumption identical to America's.
- Traditional Eskimos eat more cholesterol and saturated fats than anyone and yet have the lowest heart disease rate of any group known.
- Cholesterol is harmless unless it oxidizes. With optimal amounts of antioxidants, that process can be minimized.

CHAPTER 31

Strategies for Lowering Cholesterol

The right to search for truth implies also a duty. One must not conceal any part of what one has recognized to be true.
—Albert Einstein

One disease, many cures; many diseases, one cure.
—Chinese proverb

THE RIGHT AMOUNT OF CHOLESTEROL is needed for optimal health. Yet the high levels of free radicals in our environment increase the possibility that the cholesterol in our bloodstream may oxidize. For these and other reasons, we do not want too much cholesterol in our blood. Both high and low cholesterol increase risk to certain cancers. Just as we want the right amount of hormones, we want just the right amount of cholesterol as well. Too much and too little are equally undesirable.

People still say cholesterol is bad. Which cholesterol are they talking about?

- The cholesterol in freshly prepared animal products is harmless. If you eat more cholesterol, your liver, which naturally makes about seven eggs worth of cholesterol per day, will make less.
- The cholesterol in dried milk, aged cheese, cake mixes, or aged meats, however, should be avoided. It is oxidized and unhealthful.
- The cholesterol in your blood is fine as long as it is protected with the right antioxidants and is present in the right ratio of HDL to total cholesterol.

WHAT IS A GOOD CHOLESTEROL RATIO?

A good cholesterol ratio is the right balance of the different cholesterols in your blood. The two main forms are LDL (low-density lipoprotein) and HDL (high-density lipoprotein).

What Is a Lipoprotein?

Your body has two mediums: fatty and watery. You know from mixing salad dressings that oil and water don't mix. How do you transport the valuable fat-soluble substances that body cells need through a watery medium like blood? Build a lipoprotein, which is a package of protein, fat, and cholesterol that is assembled by the liver and circulates through the bloodstream. A lipo (fat-soluble) protein (water-soluble) is a unique molecule. It is a land and sea vehicle built for the unique task of carrying fat-soluble vitamins and other substances through watery blood.

LDL cholesterol carries more fatty acids and is more prone to oxidation. It also delivers cholesterol to the tissues. Under certain conditions it may deliver too much. For these reasons, it is called "bad" cholesterol. Yet it is not bad unless it oxidizes and is not paired with enough HDL, the "good" cholesterol. HDL cholesterol in conjunction with lecithin picks up excess cholesterol that is left by LDL. It brings it back to the liver or to tissues that need it. That is why a good cholesterol ratio is needed for optimal health.

The different densities of lipoproteins refer to the different amounts of protein they contain. Low-density cholesterol is lower in protein density, and HDL is higher in protein density. Because LDL cholesterol has more fat-soluble elements, it is more prone to damage from free radicals. The degree to which it gets damaged will depend on:

- How delicate the polyunsaturated fats are in the cholesterol molecule
- The amount and balance of antioxidants in the cholesterol molecule
- The amount of free radicals in the body

When bad eating habits, a lack of exercise, or genetics gives us too much LDL and not enough HDL, we have an undesirable cholesterol ratio and need to improve it. The right diet and nutrients along with exercise will help us do that. The ratio of HDL to total cholesterol is more important than the total amount of cholesterol in your blood. The ideal ratio of total cholesterol to HDL is 3:1.

The more stable the fats in our diet, the more stable the LDL cholesterol molecule. Virgin olive oil will remain stable in your cabinet for months. It also promotes the stability of your cholesterol when incorporated into LDL. Laboratory scientists have found it nearly impossible to oxidize LDL cholesterol made with the fatty acids from olive oil. The value of virgin olive oil comes more from its cholesterol-stabilizing effect than its cholesterol-lowering effect.

Refined polyunsaturates from the supermarket like safflower, sunflower, and corn oils are more unstable than olive oil. Commercial oil-making processes that remove antioxidants make them even more fragile. Putting them into a cholesterol molecule makes LDL cholesterol much more fragile. These commercial oils actually increase our risk of heart disease. Like a baseball catcher without his protective gear, oils that have been refined have their built-in protection removed. Their ability to promote health is lowered and the likelihood that they will damage the body is much higher. That is why it is important to consume only virgin oils made by responsible manufacturers.

WHAT IS THE RIGHT DIET FOR OPTIMAL CHOLESTEROL METABOLISM?

Studies have shown that those groups that eat a wide variety of whatever whole foods are available to them remain healthy. Their cholesterol levels, blood pressure, insulin levels, and other parameters that affect heart and artery health are excellent throughout their lives. Nutritional approaches to lowering cholesterol must put emphasis on the proven benefits of a nutrient-dense diet devoid of toxic foods. Coronary artery disease has only been found in groups that eat refined foods.

What is the best diet for lowering cholesterol? Some will do well on a high-carbohydrate, low-fat diet. Some will do better on a diet that restricts carbohydrates. Others will do better somewhere in between. The only rules are to avoid all refined foods. This includes sugar, white flour, margarine, and refined oils. It is also important to avoid overeating, lose weight if you are overweight, and to get optimal levels of all beneficial nutrients.

JUST BECAUSE IT WORKS DOESN'T MEAN IT'S THE BEST WAY TO DO IT

There are three ways to lower cholesterol:
1. Cholesterol-lowering medication.

2. The ultra-low-fat approach: no more than 20% fat for anyone; 10% or less for those with coronary artery disease; and a cholesterol intake of no more than 100 milligrams per day.
3. The nutrient-dense approach: Eat a variety of whole, unrefined foods as close to their natural state as possible. Use supplements to get optimal amounts of all beneficial nutrients. Elimination of all refined carbohydrates is paramount. Carbohydrate restriction may be necessary to lower cholesterol.

Cholesterol-Lowering Medications: Avoid Them at All Costs

Cholesterol-lowering medications are one of the greatest fiascoes of modern medicine. These medications have many side effects and significantly shorten lifespan. There has never been any proven long-term benefit from the use of cholesterol-lowering medication except in increasing the profits of the pharmaceutical industry.

The problem with cholesterol-lowering medications is that they do not address the nutrient deficiencies and toxic metal contamination that are the cause of high cholesterol levels. Cholesterol often rises as an antioxidant defense. Forcibly lowering it removes a protection system the body has set up. This can result in increased free radical damage and acceleration of diseases that are present.

Fat Restriction: A Defensive Move

Severely restricting fat can lower cholesterol. While high-carbohydrate, 10% fat diets may work, they do not address the problems caused by suboptimal nutrient intake. A lack of nutrients is implicated in causing a wide range of diseases. For those deficient in essential nutrients, there may be no choice but to restrict fat. Like a train with no tracks to run on, refined fats will derail and cause disease when part of a diet lacking in nutrients.

It may be necessary to reduce fat consumption to 10% of the diet if you:
- Do not consume enough antioxidants
- Use supermarket vegetable oils that are stripped of their nutrients
- Use white flour, sugar, and other refined carbohydrates that lack and deplete essential nutrients

While it may work, severe fat restriction is not the best approach for many. Many people who are under stress cannot maintain adequate energy levels on a diet that is high in carbohydrates and low in protein and fat. Ultra-low-fat diets high in carbohydrates can increase food cravings, decrease immune function, and negatively affect skin and hair health. Low-protein diets also do not give enough of the detoxifying protein needed by those whose elevated cholesterol is caused by toxic metals. Excess carbohydrates imbalance prostaglandins, which must be in balance for health to exist. These diets also do not balance blood sugar well. They may cause or worsen PMS and hypoglycemia. They can raise insulin levels. Insulin is one of the most reliable predictors of heart disease.

Nutrient Density and Carbohydrate Restriction

Increasing nutrient density through increasing the quality of food and the use of supplements is easier, more pleasurable and therefore, more realistic. It allows for programs that suit individual biochemistries and tastes. It also generates a greater state of overall health.

Restricting carbohydrates will lower cholesterol and triglyceride levels. Strategies for carbohydrate restriction vary from slight to severe. Some may eat as many as three to four carbohydrate servings per day, some less. A carbohydrate serving is a slice of whole-grain bread, two slices of diet whole grain bread, a half cup of cooked whole grains or whole-grain pasta, a small baked or sweet potato, or a half cup of corn, peas, or brown rice. Sugar in all forms must be avoided. Fruit must be limited to no more than two servings per day.

For the severely carbohydrate-sensitive, cholesterol levels will not get under control until carbohydrates are limited. All fruit and fruit juices may need to be eliminated, and starches may have to be limited to one or two servings per day. Work with a nutritionist to determine your individual needs.

While more research is needed, the optimal range for total cholesterol appears to be between 150 and 200.

NUTRIENTS THAT HELP BRING CHOLESTEROL INTO AN OPTIMAL RANGE

No-Flush Niacin

Inositol hexanicotinate is the preferred source of niacin for those who wish to lower their cholesterol levels. It causes no irritating flushing like regular niacin. Typical doses range between 800 and 1,600 milligrams per day with meals. Other time-released forms of niacin are not recommended. No-flush niacin will even lower cholesterol in those with familial hyper-cholesterolemia. Any high-dose niacin therapy should be supervised by your physician to make sure that niacin is not irritating your liver.

Chromium

Chromium is a very important mineral for lowering elevated cholesterol levels and for improving cholesterol ratios. Between 200 and 600 micrograms of chromium picolinate per day is very beneficial, especially when used in conjunction with niacin.

Fiber

Fiber in oat bran, psyllium husks, and flaxmeal decreases cholesterol levels. Increase consumption of all fiber-rich foods, including beans, legumes, raw nuts, fruits, and vegetables. Organic flaxmeal is the best food supplement for increasing fiber intake.

Fermented Dairy Products and Beneficial Bacteria

The Masai tribesman of Africa eat copious amounts of saturated fat. They take blood from animals and mix it with fermented milk, and yet their cholesterol levels and rates of heart disease are low. Protective factors in fermented products like yogurt appear to have a similar cholesterol-lowering effect. Certain strains of beneficial bacteria like acidophilus have also been found to lower cholesterol. Acidophilus appears to do this in two ways: It breaks cholesterol down, and it absorbs it directly. High-quality acidophilus products are recommended, preferably the refrigerated powder form.

Essential Fatty Acids

Essential fatty acids in virgin flax and canola oils have been shown to help lower cholesterol. Virtually all raw nuts have cholesterol-lowering ability. GLA in borage oil and evening primrose oil lowers cholesterol. EPA in cold-water fish and fish oils lowers triglycerides very effectively.

Vitamins C and E
Both of these vitamins have both been shown to lower cholesterol when consumed in optimal amounts.

Zinc and Copper
These trace minerals must be in balance for cholesterol metabolism to be optimal. See a nutritionist who can test you for your individual needs. A deficiency or excess of either is undesirable.

Garlic, Onions, Ginger, and Unfermented Green Tea
All four of these foods lower cholesterol.

D-limonene
This is a substance (a terpene) found in orange peel, and it inhibits one of the enzymes in the liver that makes cholesterol. It lowers cholesterol effectively and without toxicity.

Gugulipid
This herbal extract from India has been found in over twenty studies to lower cholesterol. It reduces total cholesterol, and raises HDL cholesterol as well. It is nontoxic and safe for long-term use.

CHAPTER 32

Boosting Your Immune System Naturally

I don't want to attain immortality through my work. I want to attain immortality through not dying.

—Woody Allen

O NE OF THE MOST IMPORTANT applications of nutrition is to use the right lifestyle, diet, and nutrients to keep your immune system strong. Our immune systems are under attack as never before. Our bodies are besieged by hundreds of toxic chemicals every day. We are also exposed to a myriad of bacteria, viruses, fungi, and parasites that are brought to us from all over the world due to air travel. And our immune systems do not have the supply of nutrients they once did. We are deficient and suboptimally nourished in a wide range of nutrients. This has devastating effects not only on our immune systems but on those of our children and grandchildren as well. Poor nutrition has a cumulative genetic effect.

WHAT IS THE IMMUNE SYSTEM?

The immune system is the part of the body that protects you from the constant onslaught of bacteria, viruses, and other pathogens that want to throw a party in your body. While the bone marrow, spleen, liver, thymus, lymph nodes, and white blood cells are the main players in your immune system, every part of the body—including your nervous system and mental attitude—must be in optimal health to keep your defense strong.

Antibiotics: Dangerously Abused

Antibiotics were one of the most important discoveries of the twentieth century. Like nuclear physics, however, antibiotics have enormous power which must be carefully used to benefit mankind. Unfortunately, their power has been abused. The overuse of antibiotics is creating a medical nightmare. We are close to being unable to treat many common infections. Unable to treat, that is, with drugs. The response from the pharmaceutical industry? Make new antibiotics. This does not solve the problem. It will only create more powerful and untreatable strains.

We need to attack the problem of bacterial infection from a new angle. We must take advantage of the many natural, nontoxic means available to boost the immune system. If there is a silver lining to the dark cloud of antibiotic abuse, it may be that the failure of synthetic drugs will force orthodox medicine to use nontoxic antibiotic nutrients like high doses of vitamin C. Very high amounts of vitamin A and vitamin C are some of the most potent ways to combat infections of all kinds. They do so in a way that does not create superstrains of bacteria.

PROTECTING YOUR UNIQUENESS

Each human being who was ever made is different than any other, and requires a system of recognition that protects it from all that is foreign. The cells and organs of this system do nothing but protect and maintain the uniqueness of each person. We call these cells and organs the immune system.

White blood cells roam throughout our bodies and check for a certain code on the cell membranes, like members of a club knowing a secret password. If white blood cells discover something that does not know the password, they attack it and remove it from the body. That is why organ transplant patients must have their immune systems suppressed. The body will recognize all foreign tissue and attack it.

THE IMMUNE SYSTEM PLAYERS

There are many cells that work to protect our bodies by killing pathogens like bacteria, viruses, and parasites. If there were comic books for children that told them how to stay healthy, these books would celebrate the many white blood cells that bravely defend the body:
- Macrophage Man
- B Lymphocyte Avenger
- T Lymphocyte Woman

- Natural Killer Cell Squad
- Eosinophil Crusader
- Bone Marrow Headquarters

Our superheroes need the right nutrients. Without an optimal supply of all essential nutrients accompanied by a sugar-free diet that supplies adequate protein, these defenders can no more protect you than soldiers can fight without weapons, food, and spare parts.

IMMUNE BOOSTING FOOD AND LIFESTYLE FACTORS

Avoid Sugar

What kryptonite is to Superman, sugar is to your immune cells. One dose of sugar can weaken your immune system for as long as five hours. The amount of sugar found in a sugar-sweetened soda, large glass of fruit juice, or piece of cake will stun your immune system into inaction. "Natural" sweeteners such as honey, barley malt, molasses, and maple syrup can also be immunosuppressive and should be avoided. Giving sick people ginger ale and Jell-o gives them the liquids and protein they need. It also gives them a large dose of sugar that suppresses their immune systems and prolongs illness. Stick to soups, water, sugar-free drinks such as vegetable juice, and whole, unrefined foods when trying to get well.

Barley Green and Wheat Grass

The leaves of young barley and wheat plants are an extraordinary source of immune-boosting nutrients. When they are in their grass stage, these foods are very high in beta-carotene, B vitamins, potassium, magnesium, chlorophyll, and many other nutrients. These two foods are combined with chlorella and kelp in a product known as Kyogreen. Kyogreen is a pleasant-tasting powder that dissolves instantly in water and is an easy way to give your body a powerhouse of immune-boosting nutrients. Kyogreen has been found to boost the immune system more than barley juice, wheatgrass juice, or chlorella alone. Kyogreen has also been found to have cancer-preventing properties.[459, 460]

Sunlight

Sunlight has pronounced immune-enhancing effects. It was used as a major weapon against infectious diseases in the early part of the twentieth century. Ultraviolet light has been successfully used to treat viral pneumonia, blood infections, and a range of other viral, bacterial, and fungal diseases. In 1929 the public became aware of the benefits of sunlight therapy when the King of England's health improved markedly after ultraviolet light treatment. In the 1920s and 1930s, sunlight treatment was often employed for bone tuberculosis. The discovery of penicillin in 1938 made medicine forget the sun and pushed it toward more high-tech methods of fighting disease. Twenty minutes per day appears to be the most beneficial amount, but more research is needed as our ozone layer thins.

NUTRIENTS THAT BOOST IMMUNE FUNCTION

Beta-carotene

Beta-carotene significantly boosts immune function.[461, 462, 463] Doses greater than 30 milligrams of beta-carotene per day taken for over two months dramatically enhance the immune system. This increased immune ability occurs only as long as supplements are taken.[464]

Vitamins A, C, and E

These are three of the most critical nutrients for enhancing immune function. There are hundreds of studies that show all three powerfully bolster the body's defenses. All antioxidants quench the free radicals that occur in viral or bacterial infections. This relieves the symptoms of illness and boosts the white blood cells' ability to fight off pathogens. These nutrients have been found to stimulate the immune system even in those who were not "deficient" in them.

When you have a cold, flu, or bacterial infection, your body is a battleground. The weapons that are fired are free radicals. The more free radicals are fired, the more damage to the site where the illness takes place. Taking a generous amount of these antioxidant nutrients helps prevent the damage that can occur to your body when you are ill.

B Vitamins

B vitamins are very important for many areas of immune defense. B vitamins help relax the nervous system. This is essential to the healing process. B_2 and B_6 are particularly valuable at enhancing immunity.

Magnesium

Magnesium is needed for a strong immune system. A shortage of magnesium will lower the number of white blood cells, especially T cells, resulting in weakened immunity.[465]

Zinc

Zinc is the most important mineral for the immune system. A deficiency of zinc will greatly impair the body's defenses. Low levels of zinc have been found in a large percentage of AIDS sufferers, and lead to significant decline in their immune function. Zinc supplementation has been found to be one of the most important strategies for normalizing immune function in AIDS patients.[466, 467] Zinc also helps cancer patients make more white blood cells.[468] Zinc has also been shown to significantly shorten the duration and improve the symptoms of the common cold.[469]

Selenium

Selenium is a trace mineral with powerful immune-boosting activity. Both selenium-enriched yeast and selenomethionine enhance immune function at doses of 100 to 200 micrograms per day. This immune-enhancing effect has been particularly well demonstrated in the elderly. Doses as high as 600 to 800 micrograms per day have been shown to have anti-cancer properties.[470] The full immune-stimulating effects of selenium may not be seen until six months of supplementation.[471] Exactly how selenium promotes immune function is not clear, but studies have shown that the better nourished in selenium you are, the more white blood cells you have, and the better able they are to kill invading pathogens.[472]

Glutathione

Glutathione is a protein that is one of the most important antioxidants and immune enhancers in the human body. It is found in fairly high levels in fruits and vegetables and very high levels in freshly prepared meat products. Processing of food results in a significant loss of glutathione.[473] A supplement called **NAC** (N-Acetyl Cysteine) increases the body's ability to make glutathione. Glutathione has been found to be greatly decreased in the plasma, lung fluid, and T lymphocytes of people with AIDS. This suggests that supplemental glutathione or NAC may be of great benefit to AIDS patients.[474]

Glutathione has also been shown to suppress the HIV virus in human cell cultures.[475, 476]

Taurine

Taurine is a very important amino acid for immune function. A deficiency of taurine can significantly weaken the immune system. It is found in seafood, particularly clams and other shellfish. The body makes it in small amounts. For optimal immunity, supplementation is necessary.

Ninety percent of all of the taurine in the body is in white blood cells. These cells use taurine as their battle shield as they fight off pathogens. If these defender cells do not have enough taurine, they will die in battle just as quickly as a knight without his armor. Taurine-deficient white blood cells will often not even try to defend the body, so reluctant are they to go into battle without their armor.

CoQ10

CoQ10 is a nonvitamin nutrient that has been widely studied for its ability to protect arteries, lower blood pressure, and strengthen the heart. CoQ10 is a powerful antioxidant and immune-boosting nutrient as well.

Dimethylglycine

Dimenthylglycine or DMG is an amino acid that has been found to enhance human immune function on many levels. Those who take DMG have an immune response that is up to four times greater than those who do not.[477]

Echinacea Purpurea

The roots of this plant have a well-documented ability to boost immune function. Echinacea is best used against viral infections like a cold or flu. It has also been found effective at decreasing the recurrence of chronic vaginal yeast infections by over 40%.[478] The freshly pressed juice of echinacea has been found particularly effective.[479] It should be used only for short periods of time at the onset of a cold or flu. Echinacea works by harmlessly tricking the immune system into functioning more effectively. Using echinacea as a daily supplement will significantly decrease its immunostimulating activity. Save it for when you need it. Echinacea should not be used with HIV patients or in persons with autoimmune disorders.[480]

AUTO-IMMUNE DISEASE

When a plane is flying out of control, you do not want to increase engine thrust. You want to manipulate the wing flaps and regain control of the airplane. Similarly, when someone has an autoimmune illness or a disease of immune dysfunction such as rheumatoid arthritis, HIV infection, ulcerative colitis, ankylosing spondylitis, lupus, or chronic fatigue syndrome, you do not want to stimulate all aspects of the person's immune function. Autoimmune diseases are not instances when the immune system is weak. They are diseases wherein the immune system is out of control. Autoimmunity is when the body begins to attack itself, and you do not want to stimulate all aspects of immunity under these conditions any more than you would want to give a suicidal person more guns. You first want to turn the immune system around, and wake it up from attacking the body. A cold or flu is the time to use nonspecific immunostimulants like echinacea. Autoimmune problems like those listed above are best helped by nutritional strategies that help the body regain control of itself.

The following foods and nutrients are beneficial for all kinds of immune problems, but have special value for those with autoimmune problems:

Essential Fatty Acids

Essential fatty acids are critical in helping autoimmune problems. EPA and GLA are the most therapeutically valuable fatty acids, but EFA-rich foods like flax oil can also be very helpful. These nutrients have been found effective at helping chronic fatigue, arthritis, cancer, and a range of other ailments. Many researchers believe that a deficiency of essential fatty acids may actually cause autoimmune problems.

Beneficial Bacteria

Beneficial bacteria may be helpful for all forms of autoimmune disease. Preliminary research has shown that when the GI tract is populated with unfriendly bacteria, the body may begin to attack these bacteria in a way that may also trigger it to attack other body tissues. A lack of beneficial bacteria such as acidophilus and bifidobacterium combined with an overgrowth of unfriendly bacteria is associated with many diseases. High-quality preparations of these beneficial bacteria may be some of the most important nutritional adjuncts in the prevention and treatment of many degenerative diseases, especially those that are autoimmune in nature.

Eleutherococcus Senticosus

Siberian ginseng significantly rebalances immune function. It has been studied widely for its beneficial effects in a wide range of illnesses. It enhances immune function and disease resistance in healthy subjects as well. For maximum effectiveness, standardized ginseng products are the most reliable. Eleutherococcus's unique ability to both enhance and balance the immune system may make it one of the most important botanicals for HIV-infected patients. Further study is needed.[481]

Shiitake Mushroom

Shiitakes have been shown to have marked anticancer activity. They extend the life of those with recurrent stomach, colorectal, and breast cancer. This mushroom has been studied widely for its ability to help balance and strengthen the immune system. It may have a wide range of applications in helping rebalance the immune system in conditions such as chronic fatigue, HIV infection, and other autoimmune problems.[482]

CHAPTER 33

Are There Nutritional Solutions to PMS?

E VERY MONTH OR SO, A woman's body goes through a fire drill for pregnancy. It wants to make sure the whole system works just in case the real thing happens. It is a large production, and taxes every major system in a woman's body. If there are missing nutrients, low blood sugar, yeast overgrowth, or suboptimal liver function, the ride will be a bumpy one. The result will be PMS, or premenstrual syndrome. The depression, mood swings, food cravings, cramps, and panic attacks that can be a part of PMS can make life miserable. Yet with the right diet and nutrients, PMS is often easily eliminated.

PMS is not a deficiency of antidepressant medication. It is a sign that you are missing nutrients in your diet, and you are not balancing blood sugar and metabolizing your hormones well. It is the female body crying out for a healthier diet and way of life. Give your body the healthy diet and lifestyle it needs, and you will not only eliminate PMS. You will achieve a level of health, energy, and overall wellness that you did not think possible.

Nutritional Strategies for Eliminating PMS:
- Eat adequate amounts of protein throughout the day—at least two meals with 3 or more ounces of lean meat, poultry, fish, or lentils.
- Eliminate coffee, tea, chocolate, and sodas, diet or regular.
- Remove sugar, white flour, margarines, and fried and processed foods from the diet.
- Get enough sleep.
- Exercise moderately.

- Make sure you are getting optimal amounts of all essential vitamins, minerals, and fatty acids.
- If you have a vaginal or intestinal overgrowth of yeast (candida albicans), avoid all natural sugars and repopulate your GI tract with beneficial bacteria such as bifidobacterium.
- Stop smoking and keep alcohol consumption to an absolute minimum.
- Take a special collection of nutrients known as lipotropic nutrients.

EATING ENOUGH PROTEIN

What often sets the stage for PMS is poor eating. Women who want to lose weight, particularly younger women, often eat nothing or try to exist on salads or other nutrient-poor diets. This, combined with the stress many women and young mothers are under, creates vitamin, mineral, and protein deficiencies that cause a breakdown in health we call PMS.

- Protein is of prime importance in helping the management of PMS.
- Protein eaten in moderate amounts throughout the day balances blood sugar. Unstable blood sugar creates and aggravates the mood swings of PMS.
- Protein is needed in order for the body to produce hormones that keep the female cycle functioning smoothly.
- Protein is needed for increased tissue production that takes place during the female cycle.
- The physical, mental, and emotional stress of the female cycle increases the need for protein.

IMPORTANT NUTRIENTS FOR PMS

Antioxidants

Essential for everyone, antioxidants are especially important for women with PMS. Vitamins C and E and the minerals zinc and selenium help the body balance prostaglandins, short-lived hormones that play a powerful role in the health of the woman's body. The wrong prostaglandins create the cramping associated with PMS, and antioxidants can prevent these and other symptoms. Antioxidants also enhance liver function, which is crucial to eliminating PMS.

B Complex Vitamins

These are extremely important for energy levels, hormone metabolism, liver function, and relieving bloating. Optimal amounts needed by women are in the range of 50 milligrams per day, with 400 micrograms of folic acid and 50 micrograms of B_{12}.

Magnesium

Magnesium has been found helpful in the treatment of PMS. Magnesium reduces the number of mood swings that can occur during the premenstrual period. Most women do not get enough of this valuable mineral, and should think about supplementing with at least 300 milligrams per day and taking epsom salt baths.[483]

Zinc

Zinc levels have been found to be lower in women who suffer from PMS. Zinc deficiency may lead to a decreased production of progesterone. Lowered levels of progesterone may lead to cravings for sweet and salty foods.[484] Zinc deficiency alone can contribute to decreased glucose tolerance and an increase in the craving for sweets associated with PMS.

GLA

GLA is an essential fatty acid needed for overall health. A study of forty-two women with premenstrual syndrome found that they had reduced levels of GLA and a decreased ability to manufacture it from dietary fats.[485] Without GLA, the body cannot manufacture the right balance of prostaglandins to prevent menstrual symptoms such as cramping, depression, and other problems. GLA supplements from evening primrose oil have shown to be helpful in alleviating the symptoms of PMS. Just as important, however, is to make sure that you are ingesting the nutrients needed by the body for it to make its own GLA: B complex, magnesium, vitamin C, and zinc. You also need to avoid stress and the foods that interfere with GLA production: margarine, fried foods, and junk and processed foods.

A WOMAN'S MULTIVITAMIN

Don't cheat your body with poorly made supplements that supply only the RDA levels of all nutrients. Give your body the optimal amounts it needs for PMS and for preventing degenerative diseases. When I ask most women if they take a multivitamin, they say yes. The multivitamins they are taking, however, hardly give them the optimal nutrient intake they need. If your multivitamin doesn't increase your energy and overall well-being, switch brands.

THE ESTROGEN FAMILY

The estrogen family has three members: estradiol, estrone, and estriol. Estradiol is the form that is produced by the ovaries. If estradiol is not balanced with other estrogens, the risk for cancer increases. With the right nutrients, the liver can change cancer-promoting estradiol into anticancer estriol. For these and many other reasons, it is of paramount importance to keep the liver optimally nourished.

LIPOTROPIC NUTRIENTS: A WOMAN'S SECOND MULTI

Lipotropic nutrients are a group of nutrients that support liver function and enhance the ability of the liver to metabolize hormones like estrogen. For eliminating PMS and decreasing the risk of hormone-related cancers, lipotropic nutrients are essential. Try to receive the following daily dose of these nutrients from a good lipotropic formula:

Choline	500 mg
Inositol	500 mg
B_6	50 mg
Methionine	500 mg
Magnesium	300 mg
Milk thistle extract	75 mg
Dandelion root	150 mg

SUMMING UP

Follow the principles of optimal health outlined elsewhere in this book, with special attention to eliminating sugar, consuming no more than three fruits per day, avoiding all refined carbohydrates, and eating enough protein. The female body is designed to radiate with health and energy, and will do so if you give it the nutrients and lifestyle it needs.

CHAPTER 34

Does Calcium Prevent Osteoporosis?

T O AVOID OSTEOPOROSIS YOU NEED to consume adequate amounts of calcium, yet calcium alone does not prevent the thinning of bones. Confused? No wonder. Americans have been told that calcium is the sole solution to osteoporosis. It isn't. Consuming large quantities of calcium, the chief mineral found in bone, will not strengthen them any more than eating a lot of protein will create large muscles.

Canada, the United States, Australia, France, and Scandinavian countries have the highest levels of dairy product consumption as well as the highest rates of osteoporosis. African and Asian societies have much lower rates of osteoporosis even though they consume very little calcium. How can this be?

If you have ever been to the opera, you know the enormous collaboration of talent it requires. You need great singers, an orchestra, costumes, sets, expert lighting design, and a large crew backstage to keep the whole thing running. Take any one of these elements away and even the greatest of talent will go to waste.

So it is with calcium. It is of no use to the body if all the other factors needed for strong bones are not simultaneously supplied. You need a diet balanced in all essential vitamins and minerals. You need good digestion so that you can absorb what you eat. You need to exercise. You need the right balance of hormones. And you need to stay away from sugar, white flour, and other junk foods that can undermine all of your best efforts.

START YOUNG

Imagine if you found out that when you retired you could only use the money you saved between the ages of fourteen and thirty-five. You'd be sure to save a lot during those years, wouldn't you? Although this is not true with regard to retirement funds, it does apply to the mineral stores in your bones. Adolescence and young adulthood is the most critical period for creating strong bones. By age thirty-five you achieve your peak bone mass, and from that point on you must work to maintain the bone mass that you have acquired. The higher peak bone mass you achieve, the lower your likelihood of developing osteoporosis. When you are young, you need to make sure your intake of calcium, magnesium, manganese, and all other vitamins and minerals is optimal. You will never have as much impact on your bone health as you do in your younger years, but improving nutrient intake and lifestyle habits at any age can help maintain, and in some cases improve, bone density.

Conditions that young women suffer from such as anorexia and amenorrhea can have especially negative consequences on bone health. These conditions can begin instant decline into bone weakness and should not be allowed to persist. Even frequent yeast infections impact negatively on bone health, for unfriendly bacteria in the GI tract upset female hormone metabolism. This in turn negatively affects bone growth. Because of the poor nutrition that is rampant among young women in America, many researchers believe osteoporosis actually begins in the teen years. If I could give osteoporotic women one thing, I would give them a time machine so that they could go back to their youth and lay down enough bone density to last their lifetime.

IS TOO MUCH PROTEIN THE PROBLEM?

While some studies show vegetarians have stronger bones than meat eaters, others fail to show any difference between the two groups. Several studies have shown that a high-protein diet of red meat will not increase calcium excretion. While excessive amounts of protein—more than 16 ounces of protein per day—may increase calcium excretion, diets too low in protein and high in sugar can be just as bone-weakening. Women need the right balance of protein for strong bones. Four ounces—a serving the size of a deck of cards—is a good amount of protein for most women to consume twice per day. Make sure you divide your protein throughout the day and don't eat more than 8 ounces at any meal. Higher intakes of protein will require correspondingly higher intakes of calcium and magnesium.

How Much Calcium Do We Need?

Our Stone Age ancestors had a higher peak bone mass than is found in present-day industrialized populations. They consumed between 1,500 and 3,000 milligrams of calcium per day, or roughly 2 to 3 times the U.S. RDA. They also consumed high amounts of protein, which did not negatively affect bone mass. This high intake of protein was balanced by a higher intake of minerals. This indicates that the ratio of protein to calcium may be more important than the absolute amount of each.

Some researchers have suggested that we should follow the Stone Age example and consume calcium in large quantities. Yet look at the form their calcium was in: vegetable sources that balanced calcium with a wide range of other vitamins and minerals. Their diets were also devoid of sugar and salt, both of which increase calcium excretion.

There were no dairy farms in prehistoric times. Milk is high in phosphorus, a calcium antagonist, and may not be the most effective source for calcium. Many are allergic to dairy or intolerant to the milk sugar it contains. Those countries that consume the most have high rates of osteoporosis.

Some researchers suggest all postmenopausal women should take 1,500 milligram of calcium per day. This would be fine if bones were bank accounts and calcium were money, but that is not the way it works. A wide range of nutrients is needed for healthy bones, and this calcium-as-a-drug mentality is not going to help anyone as much as a balanced intake of all nutrients would.

Few if any long-term studies have been done on large doses of supplemental calcium. Such blanket recommendations do not take into account the variations in individual biochemistry that determine calcium requirements. Some may truly need 1,500 milligrams while others would do better on 800 milligrams. The side effects of excessive calcium are numerous. They include increased plaque formation in arteries and calcification of tissues. This is never discussed by those who recommend these doses.

Once menopause has begun, estrogen levels decline, and so does bone resorption. Bone resorption is a process whereby the body recycles the calcium from dying bone cells. If bone resorption is decreasing, and the body is already wasting the calcium it has, why take more? We've seen that too much calcium is not good for us. The key is to get the calcium into your bones, not just into your bloodstream, where too much can cause problems. To get the body to use calcium correctly, you need a total nutritional, hormonal, and lifestyle approach to the problem. Due to the increased risk for certain cancers that can result from using the estradiol form of estrogen, it cannot be universally recommended as a solution. More natural, balanced estrogen formulations that contain estriol are far safer and more beneficial.

Progesterone
The most important hormone for bone health, however, is not estrogen, but progesterone. Topical progesterone cream was studied by Dr. John Lee of Sebastopol, California. One hundred postmenopausal women were given natural progesterone cream to apply for twelve consecutive days of each month for three years. They were also given supplemental calcium and vitamins C and D, were encouraged not to smoke or drink, and were told to exercise. The results were impressive: 63 of the 100 women in the study exhibited an increase in bone mass. Side effects of using natural progesterone were only positive: increase in energy and sex drive. Persons with all degrees of bone deterioration benefited remarkably from natural progesterone therapy.

Magnesium
Magnesium is also a very important mineral for bone health. Calcium cannot be laid down into bone without an adequate supply of all of the minerals needed. This includes magnesium, zinc, copper, manganese, boron, and silica. Although it only comprises .1% of bone, versus calcium, which comprises 20% of bone, magnesium plays an important role in keeping calcium from being excreted and helps the body to use calcium correctly. Some studies even point to magnesium intake as a stronger predictor of bone density than calcium intake.[486] Taking calcium in the absence of adequate magnesium and other trace minerals will only increase the amount of calcium

deposited in sites such as artery walls.[487] Magnesium deficiency may cause osteoporosis.[488] Magnesium deficiencies are common in osteoporotic patients, and low magnesium levels negatively affect estrogen metabolism. This can in turn have a weakening effect on bone mineralization.[489]

Manganese

Manganese is a trace mineral that is very important for the prevention of osteoporosis. Basketball star Bill Walton was sidelined with frequent fractures due to osteoporosis. His bone thinning was caused by a manganese deficiency. Supplements of manganese and other trace minerals reversed his condition. Most women do not get enough of this critical nutrient and could benefit from increased intake of nuts. They are a rich source of all minerals, including manganese.[490, 491, 492]

Copper

Copper is a key supplement for bone health. Studies have shown that copper levels are lower in women who suffer leg fractures. Copper is needed for the manufacture of collagen in bones. Copper supplements may prevent the fractures and mortality associated with osteoporosis. Copper levels vary widely in women, and testing by a nutritionist is recommended before supplementing with copper.[493]

Vitamin K

Vitamin K is needed to make a framework upon which all bones are built. If you don't eat enough green leafy vegetables—the only food source for vitamin K—or the beneficial bacteria in your GI tract don't make enough vitamin K, your bones will suffer. Some researchers believe that our requirements for vitamin K are higher than presently thought. Those concerned about bone health should eat as many leafy greens as possible.[494]

Those on antibiotics should increase their intake of green leafy vegetables or supplement with vitamin K. Broad-spectrum antibiotics such as tetracycline kill the beneficial bacteria that make vitamin K. Antibiotic use should always be followed by supplements of beneficial bacteria such as acidophilus and bifidobacterium. Vitamin K supplements of 100 to 500 micrograms per day are perfectly safe and may be beneficial for those who do not eat leafy greens or who undergo long-term antibiotic therapy.[495, 496, 497]

OVERALL LIFESTYLE HABITS FOR HEALTHY BONES

- Consume 800 milligrams of calcium through food and supplements every day of your life.
- Women aged twelve through twenty-four should get at least 1,000 milligrams of calcium per day through food or supplements.
- Calcium carbonate is a fine supplemental form for most women. Calcium citrate is recommended for those over fifty or those with digestive problems.
- Consume at least 400 milligrams of magnesium per day.
- Receive twenty minutes of sunshine per day.
- Exercise regularly: Dancing, walking, weight lifting, and aerobic exercise are best, but any exercise is better than none.
- Avoid sodas, regular and diet, which are both a rich source of phosphorus, which increases calcium excretion.
- Decrease intake of sugar and salt, both of which increase mineral excretion.
- Consume optimal amounts of vitamin C, folic acid, and B_6 every day.
- If you are over age forty, have a bone scan done to determine the density of your bones.
- Trace minerals such as boron, silicon, manganese, zinc, and copper are all important for healthy bones. Take an iron-free trace mineral supplement, not just calcium and magnesium.
- Avoid fluoridated water. Fluoride may displace calcium from the body and cause bones to be more brittle and likely to fracture. Use bottled or filtered water.
- Avoid aluminum baking powder, aluminum pots and pans, and anything that can increase your exposure to this toxic metal. Besides increasing risk of Alzheimer's disease, aluminum may increase the risk of osteoporosis as well. Antacids should not be used as calcium supplements, as they also may contain aluminum.
- If you are taking thyroid hormone, have your physician carefully monitor your dosage. Too much thyroid hormone may thin bones.

PART V
Weight Loss

CHAPTER 35

Weight Loss Guidelines

Distant goals are the best goals.

–Victorian saying

I MAGINE THAT IT IS THE height of the Cold War and Nikita Krushcev is meeting with the leaders of the Soviet military. "I want to conquer Kansas," he says. A stunned general asks him, "Don't you want to take over the entire nation? Perhaps invade California?" "No," he says. "We just need Kansas and the grain it has."

Pursuing weight loss alone without simultaneously aiming for optimal health is just as ridiculous. It must all come together, or it won't happen in a healthful, permanent manner. You cannot achieve long-term weight loss without examining all aspects of your health: digestion, hormonal balance, nutrient status, food allergies, mood-controlling chemicals known as neurotransmitters, emotional problems, glandular function, and genetic tendencies. It's a long list, and while we may not have the desire to look at everything that affects our health, we need to appreciate that it all comes into play when we try to lose weight. As we have seen so often, you cannot be healthy on any level without being healthy on every level.

WHAT IS WEIGHT LOSS?

Weight loss is reducing the amount of fat in your body. It is not simply weighing less or fitting into clothes better, though this should also occur. The right weight loss program should help your body hold on to as much muscle tissue as possible while stimulating fat loss. The right diet and nutrient intake combined with a moderate exercise program such as walking will help maintain lean tissue. Maintaining as much lean muscle tissue as possible is important, for it is the muscle tissue that does most of the fat burning. A higher amount of lean tissue will keep your metabolic rate elevated throughout the weight loss process and will help you keep the weight off in the long run.

The amount of your weight that is fat is your body fat percentage. The higher the percentage, the greater your risk of degenerative diseases such as heart disease, cancer, high blood pressure, and diabetes. Young men should strive for a body fat percentage of between 8% and 15%; and young women, 15% to 21%. As we age, our allowances for body fat increase gradually.

A 6-foot-3-inch, 320-pound football player with a 6% body fat percentage will not need to lose weight. He is solid muscle. The same man twenty years later, if sedentary, may be 25% fat if he kept his weight the same. He would then be in great need of reducing the amount of fat on his body. The average lifespan for a professional football player is fifty-six. Whether it is caused by increasing body fat percentage, steroid abuse, or a combination of many factors is unknown.

If at all possible, work with a nutritionist who can determine your body fat percentage. While most methods for determining body fat are reliable within a few percentage points, electrical impedance testing is not recommended. It is not reliable.

Do Diets Work?

When people say diets don't work, I don't know what they mean. Perhaps they mean that fad or restrictive diets are not effective for long-term weight loss. This is often true, because the wrong things are being restricted. Fat and protein are usually limited, and a liberal consumption of carbohydrates is recommended. Often, this is the opposite of what needs to be done. Most overweight women eat too many carbohydrates and do not get enough protein, essential fatty acids, and other essential nutrients. If mechanics put the engines of cars in backward after fixing them, we wouldn't say, "Cars don't work." We would say, "Mechanics are inept." When I hear people say, "Diets don't work," I want to say, "No, diet counselors are inept."

Diet comes from the Latin word *diaeta* meaning "a way of life." Diets will only work when they suit your metabolism and lifestyle. Poorly designed weight loss programs, tried in a hit-

or-miss style, are usually ineffective. Correctly designed diets created by qualified health professionals to suit individual metabolisms are very effective.

THERE IS NO SUCH THING AS FATTENING FOOD

Are peanuts fattening? Is bread fattening? These are unanswerable questions. There is no food with an absolute effect that is the same on everyone. We all have different metabolisms. You might as well ask, "Does a trumpet sound good in a symphony?" Yes, when it plays the right melody at the right time. But if it plays when it is not supposed to, it will sound awful. That is how food comes together in our diet: Balanced with other whole foods, virtually any food that is not refined can have a place in our diet, as long as it is combined with an assortment of other nutrient-dense foods in a well-planned menu.

There are no fattening foods. There are only fattening metabolisms. Your body's hormones and enzymes will decide whether the food you eat will turn into fat. The following factors influence how well we will burn off the food we eat:

- Thyroid hormone levels
- Insulin levels
- Growth hormone levels
- Amount of muscle tissue
- Tissue responsiveness to hormones like insulin and thyroid hormone
- Number of fat-burning mitochondria in your muscle cells
- Levels of nutrients needed for fat burning

WHAT TO ASK ABOUT FOOD

When most people look at a food label, the first two things they ask are:

- How many calories does it have?
- How much fat does it have?

These factors are not as important as the hormonal effects of food. More calories and more fat may cause weight gain, but they do not always. Choosing foods because of their fat and calorie content is like making friends on the basis of IQ or income levels. You choose your friends because of their overall effect on your life, not because of their salary. Select foods for their overall effects as well, and look beyond numbers like calorie or fat content.

When considering eating any food, you should ask only one question:

What effect will this food have on my metabolism?

Often, what keeps us from understanding nutrition is not that we lack the right answers but that we ask the wrong questions. By merely looking at the calorie and fat content of food, we miss the much larger issue of food's metabolic and hormonal effect on the body. This is not to say that fat and calorie content are insignificant; they are not. Too many calories and too much fat is undesirable. Yet calorie and fat content are less significant than the hormonal reaction that all foods cause. It is these hormonal results that will decide whether the effect of food on our body will be positive or negative. It is a lack of understanding of this hormonal effect of food that keeps many people from losing weight.

The Hormonal Effect of Food
In 1982 the Nobel Prize was given to scientists who made groundbreaking discoveries about prostaglandins, a powerful class of hormones that control the body. The most powerful effect foods have on your body is their effect on these hormones and hormones like insulin. When Julius Caesar sat on his throne, thumbs up saved the life of a prisoner, and thumbs down meant death. That supreme power is wielded over weight loss by hormones like insulin and prostaglandins. If insulin levels are high or prostaglandins are imbalanced, weight loss can be difficult if not impossible. What upsets prostaglandins and insulin the most are missing nutrients, a lack of essential fatty acids, and consumption of refined carbohydrates, especially sugar, which triggers insulin to store fat. Even too many unrefined carbohydrates, like beans and brown rice, can raise insulin, imbalance prostaglandins, and make weight loss nearly impossible.

If only eating fat made you fat, then why did Americans gain weight between 1978 and 1990 even though they ate less fat as a percentage of total calories? The food they ate—high in sugar and low in nutrients—made their hormones store more fat. When 26,473 Americans were studied, it was found that those who ate the most nuts were the least obese. The more fat they ate, the less fat they were.[498] This goes against all conventional wisdom, but fits the hormonal model of weight loss and weight gain perfectly. Nuts are high in fat—a high-quality, beneficial fat. Nuts stabilize blood sugar, lower cholesterol, lower blood pressure, and provide satiety. They also provide the nutrients and essential fatty acids needed to create the right prostaglandins that stimulate weight loss. Fat-free cookies may have little fat and fewer calories than nuts, but the sugar in them will raise insulin, imbalance blood sugar, stimulate your appetite, upset prostaglandins, and raise cholesterol. You may be allergic to the wheat in the cookies, and that may make you even more tired and can also stop weight loss. Think of food in three-dimensional terms, not just according to the statistics on the label.

If you could control the actions of the hormones in your body, you could eat all the food you want and still lose weight. When you put together a nutrition program for weight loss, therefore, you want to select the foods that will help create the right hormonal balance.

Exercise and Hormonal Balance
Much of the benefit of exercise for weight loss comes from its ability to help lower insulin levels and to promote insulin to work more effectively:

- Insulin levels are lowered during and after exercise. This increases weight loss.
- Exercise stimulates the tissues of the body to respond more effectively to insulin.
- By increasing insulin sensitivity of muscle tissues, exercise helps balance blood sugar and eliminate cravings.
- By increasing insulin response from the muscle tissues, exercise stimulates more muscle growth. Higher muscle mass increases metabolic rate and promotes weight loss.

Exercise has other benefits important to the weight loss process. Exercise puts more oxygen in the body, which is needed for fat burning. Exercise also stimulates the detoxification of the body, which is important during weight loss. Don't end your exercise with a sugar- or fruit-juice-sweetened drink, or you will diminish the hormonal benefits of aerobic activity.

The Best Diet for Hormonal Balance and Weight Loss

The most effective way to keep insulin and prostaglandins favorably balanced for weight loss is to consume a diet that contains nearly equal amounts of protein, fat, and carbohydrates. Researchers like Dr. Barry Sears have suggested that the ideal diet for weight loss should have a ratio of 40% carbohydrates, 30% fat, and 30% protein. Others, like Dr. Gerald Reaven, feel that even less carbohydrates may be desirable. Individual requirements will vary. In the end, all of our science brings us back to what our grandmother knew: A balanced diet is best.

CHAPTER 36

Which Supplements Help Weight Loss?

NUTRITIONAL TUNE-UP

When your car isn't running well, you bring it in for a tune-up. You can't ignite gas without good spark plugs. The same thing is true with the cells of your body. Without the right vitamins, minerals, and essential fatty acids, you cannot burn fats and sugars and turn them into energy. Optimal combustion of food is critical to the weight loss process.

Also, when your car needs a tune-up, you don't fix it by driving it five hundred miles. Neither can the many problems caused by the nutrient deficiencies commonly seen in over-weight people be solved through exercise. You need to give the body the right nutrients and a diet that will balance hormones first and foremost. Exercise is an important adjunct to weight loss, and some will not lose weight until they incorporate it. But it is not as important as eating a hormone-balancing diet that contains all nutrients beneficial to the weight loss process.

A list of beneficial supplements for weight loss follows. This is a general discussion not meant to prescribe specifically for anyone. Each person has completely different needs. The only absolute recommendation that can be made for anyone trying to lose weight, whether they ten pounds or over a hundred, is to take antioxidants.

Antioxidants are essential for protecting the body during weight loss. As we release fat from our fat cells, we also liberate the toxic chemicals that the body stores in them. The body protects the nervous system and other delicate tissues from the damage of mercury, dioxin, and other neurotoxins by putting them in fat cells. Once liberated, these chemicals can cause irritation and damage to many tissues in the body, particularly the liver. In order to help detoxify these damaging substances, the body requires the following antioxidants:

Vitamin C	1–2 grams
Vitamin E	100–400 IUs
Zinc Picolinate	15–50 mg per day
Selenium	100 mcg per day
N-Acetyl Cysteine (NAC)	1,000 mg per day
Standardized Milk Thistle Extract	150 mg per day

It is best to work with a degreed nutritionist or nutritionally oriented physician familiar with the use of nutritional supplements if you yourself are not. NAC should not be taken by diabetics as it can block insulin receptors.

One of the many reasons commercial weight loss programs often fail and are unsafe is that they do not adequately detoxify their clients. Toxins that are released during weight loss cannot only damage tissues, they can cause depression or other undesirable moods. This may be one of the reasons dieters abandon most weight loss programs, because going off the diet will stop the release of toxins that cause depression or other mood changes. One of the reasons water fasting is particularly discouraged is that it stimulates the release of a great deal of toxic material without any of the detoxifying nutrients to help manage the increased oxidative load. Detoxification should precede or accompany every weight loss program to minimize the damage that free radicals can cause. The UltraClear program, available through health professionals, is an excellent nutritional approach to detoxifying the body.

Fiber

Fiber is a very important element for weight loss, whether through food or supplemental foods like organic flaxmeal, guar gum, oat bran, or other sources. Fiber provides a sense of fullness, and balances energy levels. This is especially true for those on low-carbohydrate diets who have reduced their intake of fiber-rich starchy grains, beans, and fruits.

Vitamin C

Vitamin C is needed for weight loss detoxification and for thyroid hormone formation, the most important hormone needed for weight loss and metabolic regulation. Vitamin C is also needed for the body to make carnitine, another substance needed for fat burning. Three grams of vitamin C per day has been found to encourage weight loss even without calorie restriction.[499]

Chromium Picolinate

This is a nutrient that has been studied widely for its ability to help the body burn fat and sugar more effectively. Most dieters find 200 to 600 micrograms per day helpful.

Iron

Iron is needed in adequate amounts for weight loss. Iron is needed for the body to make carnitine. Iron deficiency also decreases your body's ability to make thyroid hormone. A lack of iron can lower body temperatures, a sign of decreased fat burning. Iron-deficient women supplemented with 78 milligrams of iron for twelve weeks increased their thyroid hormone levels and body temperatures, demonstrating an increase in metabolism.[500] Menstruating women may need iron when trying to lose weight, especially if they are avoiding animal products. Fatigue comes from many sources, and does not automatically signal an iron deficiency. A serum ferritin test will indicate whether iron is needed.

Zinc

Zinc is a very important adjunct to the weight loss process. Zinc is another valuable mineral that helps sensitize tissues to the effects of insulin, and in so doing, helps to minimize cravings. It also helps insulin do its job of encouraging sugar burning and lean muscle growth, both of which help weight loss.

Selenium

Selenium, as we have seen, is important for the detoxification process that must accompany weight loss. Selenium is also needed for activation of thyroid hormone.[501] Selenium supplementation in selenium deficient hypothyroid patients should always be accompanied by iodine supplementation.[502, 503]

Carnitine

Carnitine is a nonvitamin nutrient that acts like a forklift, transporting fatty acids to the part of the cell that burns them off. For this reason, carnitine has become a popular nutrient for weight loss and for those who want to lower their body fat levels. It is manufactured by the body from the amino acids lysine and methionine, with the help of vitamin C, iron, B3, and B_6. Red meat, especially lamb, is the most prominent source of carnitine in the diet. Vegetarian dieters may have a particular need to supplement with carnitine.

Although the body can make carnitine, it may not always be able to keep up with increased demands for this nutrient that the body can have during weight loss. This is especially true on low-protein diets or when the diet lacks the cofactor nutrients listed above.[504, 505] Carnitine is needed at optimal levels for weight loss to occur in some individuals, especially in slow metabolisms and when there is low thyroid function. It is especially indicated for those on low-carbohydrate diets. Helpful doses range between 500 and 2,000 milligrams per day. Start with small amounts and take it in the morning before breakfast. You should feel an increase in energy and see improved weight loss.

CoEnzyme Q10

This is a nutrient that has been found to enhance immune function, cardiac function, and is increasingly suspected of being deficient in those who are obese. Some studies show half of the overweight population may be in need of CoQ10 to lose weight efficiently. Doses range from 25 to 75 milligrams per day. Persons with heart disease should use CoQ10 under the supervision of their health-care professionals, as CoQ10 benefits heart function and can decrease the need for certain medications.

Flaxseed Oil

The right fats are essential for healthy weight loss. Your body cannot produce the hormones necessary to lose weight without essential fatty acids present in foods like flaxseed and canola oils. Failing to eat these foods during a weight loss program is a common mistake, and can create imbalances in the body that may make weight loss difficult. Dry skin is a common sign of essential fatty acid deficiency. While it is true that fat contains more calories, a lack of the right fats will keep you from burning calories.

GLA

GLA is a fatty acid that helps stimulate fat burning in the body. It is made by the body from fats such as safflower, sunflower, and corn oils. But if you lack the magnesium, zinc, B vitamins, and other nutrients and enzymes needed to make it, or you are consuming margarine, alcohol, sugar, or other refined foods, you may not make enough and may need to supplement. There is evidence that persons with low thyroid function have trouble making their own GLA and are in need of supplementation. Food sources of GLA are evening primrose oil, black-currant seed oil, and, by far the most economical source, borage oil. Individual requirements vary widely. Some may need only one 1,000-milligram borage oil capsule per day, while others will need three. Still others will only do well on the more expensive evening primrose oil, anywhere from two to ten capsules per day with meals.

Brindall Berry

Garcinia cambogia is a fruit popular in India. It contains a compound known as HCA (hydroxycitrate), which may be helpful for those trying to lose weight. HCA appears to inhibit an enzyme the body uses to make fat. HCA not only limits fat storage, but increases fat burning. When the body cannot store fat, it has more opportunity to burn it off. Human studies have confirmed that an extract of brindall berry can be valuable when integrated into a weight loss program. In one study, those taking 500 milligrams of brindall berry extract three times per day lost eleven pounds in three months, while those not taking it lost an average of four.[506, 507] Because it encourages the liver to make more sugar, diabetics should probably not use brindall berry.

Spices

Herbs and spices are a source of trace minerals and flavonoids valuable to the weight loss process. Cinnamon, cloves, fenugreek, and other spices contain trace minerals and other substances that help the body balance blood sugar more effectively. Virtually all herbs and spices are a rich source of flavonoids and other substances that are very powerful antioxidants that are needed to protect the liver from free radicals. Bioflavonoids have also been shown to help reduce the amount of heavy metals and other toxins in the body. They also increase the flavor and enjoyment of meals. This is important during weight loss, when meals are often needlessly boring and bland.

Pleasure

Pleasure is the most important nutrient in any weight loss program. Diet programs fail for many reasons; one of them is that they leave dieters starving for enjoyment they are used to getting from the food they eat. If you do not enjoy food, you may deprive yourself to the point that you throw your whole weight loss project out the window. It is important to use all of the senses that have been designed to help you enjoy food, or your body will revolt.

Helpful strategies include:

- Eating out at a good restaurant twice per month, budget permitting. Have normal serving sizes and a not-too-sweet dessert.
- Using spices and flavoring agents more liberally on food, especially if it is a lower-fat version of your favorite food.
- Having small amounts of your favorite food now and then, no matter what it is.

CHAPTER 37

Top Ten Ways to Stop Cravings

I can resist anything except temptation.

—Oscar Wilde

1. **Eat enough protein.** Snack on raw almonds, low-fat cheese, sugar-free yogurt, or leftover chicken. Small amounts of protein throughout the day are the single best strategy for balancing blood sugar and energy levels and eliminating cravings.

2. **Supplement with trace minerals.** Make sure to get enough zinc picolinate and chromium picolinate, which balance blood sugar by helping insulin work more effectively.

3. **Use herbs and spices** liberally for added flavor and for the blood-sugar-balancing effects they have.

4. **Check for candida.** Make sure you do not have an overgrowth of candida albicans in the GI tract. A low-carbohydrate diet combined with high-quality refrigerated acidophilus and bulgaricus products may be helpful.

5. **Avoid foods that you may be allergic or intolerant to.** Common offenders include wheat and all wheat-containing foods, milk and dairy products, and others. Often the food you crave most is the one you are allergic or intolerant to.

6. **If you crave chocolate, try magnesium.** Chocolate is more than delicious; it is a rich source of magnesium, which most people lack. A deficiency in magnesium may trigger chocolate cravings. I have seen supplements of magnesium of 500 milligram per day and/or epsom salt baths help relieve chocolate cravings.

7. **Avoid sugar** in all forms, which triggers unstable blood sugar levels and increases cravings.

8. **Standardized panax ginseng extract** can be very helpful at boosting energy levels and balancing blood sugar, both of which are needed to eliminate cravings.

9. **Use flaxseed oil.** If you are craving fatty foods, increase your intake of essential fatty acids through foods like flax, walnut, and canola oils.

10. **Exercise.** Moderate aerobic exercise decreases cravings by helping tissues respond better to insulin, and by increasing the level of free fatty acids in the blood that can be used for energy.

PART VI

Aggressive Preventive Medicine

CHAPTER 38

How to Find a Good Nutritionist

People can have any color car they want so long as it is black.
—Henry Ford

I MAGINE IF, WHEN LINDBERG FLEW to Paris in 1927, only a handful of reporters were there to meet him, and the story remained buried in the back pages of newspapers, with articles entitled "Did He Really Do It Alone, Or Was He Helped?" That is the greeting that optimal nutrition is getting from most dietitians. The past twenty years has witnessed an avalanche of scientific data that confirms aggressive nutritional strategies can reduce the rate of many degenerative diseases. And yet the people with the most potential for implementing this exciting information—dietitians—are not interested.

We are told to be excited about the Hubble Telescope, which certainly has helped us understand space better. But it is a candle in the sun in importance compared to the relevant information that has been put together over this first century of nutrition. We are told we need more studies, yet if we only implemented what we already know, we could significantly reduce the rates of degenerative disease in America. Dietitians are, as a group, not interested in optimal health, only adequate health, which isn't really adequate at all. The American diet has problems that are not solved by eating less fat and eating more vegetables. Such a strategy is about as effective as rearranging the deck chairs on the *Titanic*.

A GOOD NUTRITIONIST IS HARD TO FIND

Like a prospector's pan, the world of dietitians is a murky one filled with specks of gold. Occasionally you find an R.D. who understands how to use therapeutic nutrition to encourage

263

optimal health in his or her clients. Yet they are the exception, not the rule. Dietitians can be intelligent, but are rarely open-minded and usually cannot see beyond the boundaries of their own incomplete training.

I often think of how much more dietitians would enjoy their careers if they were trained in helping people achieve the highest levels of health possible instead of merely working to keep people alive.

If dietitians were taught everything that nutrition could do therapeutically, the need for physicians would be greatly reduced. Whether they know it or not, the dietitians who frown on the use of supplements are holding back their entire profession.

In the future, there should be a new health-care technician known as the dietitian practitioner. This would be someone who would have at least two more years training than standard dietitians. They would have the ability to treat blood pressure, digestive, immune, and other nutrition-related disorders with diet, supplement, and lifestyle changes. It would take a great burden off the beleaguered physicians, who do not do such a good job with these ailments anyway. It would also greatly reduce the cost of health care. There would be more time for patient supervision and education, and a much greater chance of long-term success. In certain ailments, nutrition should be the therapy of first choice. We need better-trained dietitians to help manage these conditions.

LOOKING FOR A NUTRITIONIST

The most important quality a nutritionist should have is strong clinical experience. Whether you are trying to lose weight, lower your cholesterol, or deal with any other nutrition-related problem, ask your prospective nutritionist, "Have you ever dealt with anyone who has had this problem before? What is your success rate?"

Another important aspect of your interaction with a nutritionist is an explanation of why you are being put on a particular diet or why certain nutritional supplements are being recommended. Ideally, you and your nutritionist should review summaries of studies. One of the best books that provides a wide range of summaries is *Nutritional Influences on Illness*, by Melvin Werbach, M.D., published by Third Line Press. It contains thousands of studies organized in alphabetical order according to each particular ailment. It clearly demonstrates the value of nutritional support in a wide range of illnesses. It should be on every nutritionist's desk.

Choosing Wisely

Before you make an appointment with a nutritionist, interview him or her over the phone. Use the scoring method below to help you make your decision.

Ask your nutritionist:

What kind of degree do you have?

Registered dietitian	_____	+ 5
Bachelor's degree in nutrition	_____	+ 5
Master's degree in nutrition	_____	+ 10
Ph.D. in nutrition	_____	+ 15
Degree in naturopathic medicine	_____	+ 15

What kind of diets do you design?

Everyone is put on a high-carbohydrate, low-fat diet.	_____	− 10
Each person is given a diet to suit his or her own unique bio-chemistry.	_____	+ 10
White flour products are permitted.	_____	− 10
Margarine is recommended.	_____	− 10
Can I have phone numbers of some of your happy clients to call?	_____	+ 10 if "yes"
Do you look for nutrient levels through hair and blood tests?	_____	+ 10 if "yes"
Do you think most people need supplements?	_____	+ 15 if "yes"
How many nutrients does the body require? (roughly 45)	_____	+ 10 if correct

Scoring

20 or below: Nutrition from the Eisenhower era. Avoid.

20–45: You can do better.

Above 50: Make an appointment. This nutritionist will be able to help you.

Ask your prospective nutritionist, "Which recent finding in nutrition most excited you?" A good nutritionist will follow the latest research like a stockbroker follows the stock market. Someone who doesn't have an answer to this question should be avoided. A nutritionist unfamiliar with the most recent information will not give you the best of care.

CHAPTER 39

Top Ten Reasons Why Most Doctors Do Not Know Anything About Nutrition

1. **They are not taught it in medical school.**

2. **Drug company salespeople provide most of the continuing education for the modern physician's clinical practice.**

3. **Using nutrition as a healing and preventive modality takes time.** Physicians are drowning under paperwork and the many pressures of maintaining a busy practice. Teaching their patients how to use diet and lifestyle to get healthy takes time they either don't have or don't want to give.

4. **Most physicians want to practice "politically correct" medicine.** They do not want to get a reputation among their colleagues as being a "nutrition nut." They may lose referrals and encounter other problems from the local medical board and the FDA, which does not like physicians who admit that nutrients can affect your health.

5. **Most physicians think nutrition is "wimpy."** They use drugs that may effect one enzyme system and scoff at nutrients like magnesium, which is needed for three hundred enzymes.

6. **Nutrition promotes the self-empowerment of the patient, which some physicians find threatening.** Nutrients that promote health do not require a prescription, and can be obtained indefinitely without an office visit.

7. **Physicians are afraid of suggesting therapies that could not be defended as normal, orthodox medicine in case something goes wrong.**

8. **Surgery, chemotherapy, and other invasive procedures are very profitable.** Switching to less invasive approaches means a significant loss of income.

9. **Many patients come to the doctor expecting to be given a prescription.** They do not want to make diet and lifestyle changes. If they do not receive a drug as a solution, they will go elsewhere.

10. **René Descartes.** The systematic approach to modern science that Descartes instigated in the seventeenth century has led to many advances, but it has also encouraged a compartmentalized, mechanical view of the human body. This has led to a medical system of specialists who know more and more about less and less. Nutrition is by its very nature holistic, for it affects the body as a whole. The very foundation of the training of physicians is a systematic understanding of the body that is antiholistic, and therefore antinutrition.

CHAPTER 40

Aggressive Preventive Medicine

He who lets the world, or his own portion of it, choose his plan of life for him, has no need of any other faculty than the ape-like one of imitation. He who chooses his plan for himself, employs all his faculties. He must use observation to see, reasoning and judgment to foresee, activity to gather materials for decision, discrimination to decide, and when he has decided, firmness and self-control to hold to his deliberate decision.

—John Stuart Mill, *On Liberty*

The only thing I don't regret are my mistakes.

—Oscar Wilde

BELOW CHEYENNE MOUNTAIN IN COLORADO sits one of America's main defense installations. It operates around the clock, gathering information from sensing devices all over the world. With pinpoint accuracy, it lets us know where virtually every enemy ship, troop, and major weapon is located up to the second. We know instantly the moment our security is threatened.

A senator in Washington thinks this is a waste of money. He says our shores have not been attacked in half a century. He wants to eliminate the satellites that gather information, the submarines that act as invisible deterrents, and the carriers that patrol the seas. "Military bases along each coastline to defend us are all we really need," he says. Yet it is this aggressive approach that has kept the peace for the past half century, and this same aggressive preventive approach to degenerative diseases must be employed if we are going to get America healthy.

We need to be as aggressively protective of our health as we are of our freedom. Our military makes it extremely difficult for anyone to start a conflict. Our medicine must make it very difficult for degenerative disease processes to begin as well.

And just as the military, intelligence, and diplomatic corps stay watchful of the balance of power in distant lands, we, too, must be concerned about soil erosion, water pollution, the use of pesticides, toxic creations of the chemical industry, the thinning of the ozone layer, and the destruction of rain forests. We must be watchful over our global village both politically and biochemically. Collapsing foreign rain forests affect us as much as collapsing foreign governments. They begin an ecological domino effect.

Aggressive preventive medicine would employ strategies along the following lines:

- All children would be told about the negative effects of foods like white flour, sugar, hydrogenated oil-laden junk foods, refined oils, and fried foods. They would understand them not as "forbidden foods," but foods that they should avoid if they want to be healthy.
- Doctors would make sure all patients had an optimal intake of all essential nutrients, particularly antioxidants, trace minerals, and essential fatty acids. Testing would determine individual needs.
- Physicians would check their patients for adequate digestive function, and would suggest consumption of fermented dairy products and supplements of beneficial bacteria on a regular basis.
- Patients' blood would be routinely tested for a dangerous protein byproduct known as homocysteine. If elevated, B complex vitamins would be used to lower homocysteine.
- Everyone over age fifty would be on a high-quality ginkgo preparation to maximize circulation, quench free radicals, and optimize brain health.
- Functional tests would examine the liver to make sure that it is not only free of disease, but is detoxifying at an optimal level. Patients who work in an office with many chemicals in the air, who breathe smog, or who drink alcohol would be given a supplement of standardized milk thistle extract to enhance liver health.
- Anyone with a family history of diabetes would be given optimal amounts of niacinamide, chromium, and essential fatty acids from a very young age.
- All women would be given a nutritional program that would help enhance the ability of the liver to metabolize carcinogenic estrogen (estradiol) into its less carcinogenic form (estriol).

- A physician would begin a visit with his or her patient with the question "So where are you getting your forty-five nutrients?"
- The surgeon general would issue warnings on junk foods, like:

Warning: This food contains hydrogenated oils, which the surgeon general has determined raise cholesterol, cause heart disease, and may be involved in the development of other degenerative diseases.

Warning: This food is high in refined sweeteners, which the surgeon general has determined suppress immune function, deplete nutrients, and cause a wide variety of degenerative diseases.

JUNK FOOD TAX

Diets low in nutrients and high in white flour, sugar, hydrogenated oils, and refined flours cause disease. If we were to put a tax on these foods, the money collected could be used to pay for all the diseases they cause. It is not fair that those of us who do not eat destructive foods bear the health-care costs of those who do. There are many Americans who care more about their pocketbooks than their health, and perhaps such a tax would give them more incentive to eat health-promoting foods.

The most extraordinary thing about modern medicine is that it doesn't operate from a model of wellness. It trains physicians to diagnose and eradicate disease, not generate health. No one would argue that physicians must know how to diagnose and treat illness. But most Americans do not have an acute disease; most are chronically unwell. They are wandering in a dangerous gray territory where they can slowly develop many serious degenerative problems. By the time they see a physician, prevention is no longer possible, and heroic intervention with drugs or surgery may be needed. Instead of counseling people on how to improve their diet and lifestyle to prevent clogged arteries, we wait for arteries to clog and graft a leg vein across the heart. The public regards this operation as lifesaving, but it is really the end result of irresponsible medicine. The patient and often the doctor should be blamed for allowing arteries to clog to a life-threatening degree.

A brilliant diagnostician is nowhere near as valuable as someone who prevents illness. The medical profession encourages and rewards those who specialize. Though specialists are needed, we have an incomprehensibly larger need for the preventive foot soldier, whether in the form of an enlightened dietitian or nutritionally oriented physician. Everyone in the health-care system must view the generation of optimal health — not the treatment of acute disease — as the most important job.

The steam engine was invented in the first century A.D. by the Roman inventor Hero of Alexandria, yet it was not until James Watt reinvented it in the seventeenth century that it was actually employed for the benefit of mankind. Roman society had no interest in harnessing Hero's curiosity for practical applications. Will optimal nutrition suffer the same fate? Will we harness its power? Or will it remain something of a curiosity, of interest only to a subset of the population called "health nuts?"

ARE WE BEING TOO CONSERVATIVE?

We didn't do long-term studies on atomic weapons before using them to end World War II. We acted decisively with the information at hand. Waiting would have cost more American lives. The same decisiveness is needed to solve the health-care crisis in America, and the bomb we want to drop is optimal health. Although we may never achieve optimal health for everyone, we must have it as our goal if we hope to see any decrease in the rates of degenerative disease.

While leaving a concert of his work in Los Angeles, composer Igor Stravinsky was complimented by a fan who came up to him and said, "Mr. Stravinsky, your music is too good!" "No," Mr. Stravinsky said, "never be too good. Only be good enough."

Hopefully modern medicine will risk being too good. It's a risk we have to take.

CHAPTER 41

Real Food, Fake Food

I F YOU GET CONFUSED ABOUT nutrition, just remember that you should eat food as close to its natural state as possible. Avoid junk foods. They are low in nutrients, are often high in sugar, and have other toxic ingredients added to them as well. Don't eat foods for what they don't have. Even a Twinkie can be cholesterol-free. Eat real, whole, unrefined foods for what they do have: a rich array of nutrients that promote health.

Whole grains are far better than white "enriched" flours and pastas that have had the vast majority of their nutrients removed.

Real fruit is better than dried fruit or fruit juice. Real fruit has vitamins, minerals, beneficial phenolic compounds, essential fatty acids, and many other valuable substances not found in refined fruit products. Pureed fresh fruit is always better than white sugar, honey, fruit juice concentrate, or any other concentrated sweetener.

Fresh vegetables are always better and have more vitamins and minerals than those that are canned or frozen.

Virgin oils in opaque containers, such as virgin flaxseed, canola, and olive oil, are health-promoting. Refined supermarket vegetable oils and hydrogenated oils cause disease.

Freshly prepared meats are better than ground, smoked or aged meats. Aged meat or meat that has been ground days ahead of time often has disease-causing oxidized cholesterol that is rarely found in fresh meat. If you want to consume ground meats such as hamburger, buy the lowest-fat cut of meat you can and have it ground right before using. Completely avoid all aged meats, including aged steaks and sausages.

Fresh seafood is better than that which has been canned or smoked. The fresher the fish, the more intact its valuable fatty acids will be.

Raw nuts and seeds are health-promoting; oil-roasted nuts and seeds that have added salt can diminish health and cause degenerative disease.

Herbs and spices are better than artificial colorings and flavorings.

Raw, certified milk is better than homogenized, pasteurized milk.

Butter is better than margarine.

Fresh eggs are rich in beneficial nutrients and are far better than chemical-laden egg substitutes.

Unfermented green tea is far richer in beneficial compounds than tea that has been processed into regular black tea. Unfermented green tea is a much better drink than coffee.

Nutritional supplements are also essential to bring our intake of nutrients to an optimal level. Even the most carefully selected diet cannot supply optimal amounts of vitamins and minerals. Everyone should—at the very least—take a high-quality iron-free multivitamin, as well as 1,000 milligrams of vitamin C and 200 IUs of vitamin E every day.

Appendix

I F YOU ARE IN THE New York City or Fairfield County, Connecticut area and are looking for a nutritionist, you could do no better than to contact the many fine nutritionists who work with me at Designs for Health. They are the only group in the country that I know of that is thoroughly trained in the principles of optimal health. You can reach me or one of the excellent nutritionists I work with at:

Robert Crayhon, M.S.
1-B Quaker Ridge Road
Suite #432
New Rochelle, N.Y. 10804
(914) 632-4565

ALTERNATIVE MEDICINE FOR TOTAL HEALTH

Each week, I interview innovators in the field of medicine and nutrition on my national cable TV show, "Alternative Medicine for Total Health." Every Saturday, my guests and I discuss the latest ways to prevent disease and heal the body using nutrition and other wellness strategies. At the time of printing, the show can be seen nationwide Saturdays from 7:00 to 7:30 P.M. Eastern Time. It can also be picked up by satellite viewers at the same time on G3, Channel 6. Check local listings or ask your local cable operator to carry this exciting show. Write to the address above if you have trouble finding it.

TOTAL HEALTH MAGAZINE

If you are interested in the latest findings in nutrition, I recommend a subscription to *Total Health* magazine. I have three regular columns in it and also serve as associate editor. It boasts contributions from the finest physicians, herbalists, exercise experts and other researchers who give you cutting-edge health information. I answer reader questions in every issue. Subscriptions are inexpensive. Published six times yearly.

Total Health
165 North 100 East, Suite 2
St. George, UT 84770
(800) 788-7806

PUBLICATIONS FOR THE ADVANCED READER

For health professionals or advanced students of nutrition, all of the following resources are highly recommended. Whether you are a health professional new to nutrition, or are a nutritionist who has been in practice many years, all of these carefully chosen resources will help expand your knowledge tremendously. I find all of them extremely valuable.

The Journal of Optimal Nutrition
Brian Leibovitz, Ph.D., Editor
2552 Regis Drive
Davis, CA 95616
(916) 756-3311
Fax (916) 758-7444
The Journal of Optimal Nutrition is the only journal to focus the benefits of nutrients in optimal amounts. *JON*'s editorial board boasts some of the most respected physicians and nutrition researchers from around the world. Highly recommended for health-care professionals and all students of nutrition.

The Townsend Letter
911 Tyler Street
Port Townsend, WA 98368-6541
(360) 385-6021
Self-described as "An Informal Newsletter for Doctors Communicating to Doctors," The Townsend Letter's ten yearly issues are three hundred pages of interesting information on all areas of complementary medicine. A must for health-care practi-

tioners or anyone interested in the progress of nutritional medicine.

Tree Farm Communications
23703 NE Fourth Street
Redmond, WA 98053
(800) 468-0464
Find out what the latest researchers are saying. Listen to Tree Farm's extensive library of taped talks from the most important seminars on nutrition and complementary medicine, sports medicine, naturopathy, etc. Contact them for their latest free catalog.

Health Realities
Queen and Company
P.O. Box 49308
Colorado Springs, CO 80949-9308
(800) 414-3438
Health Realities is the most informative and carefully researched nutrition newsletter I've ever seen. It comes out approximately four times per year and covers the latest findings in nutrition and how it can be integrated into medical practice. Recent issues featured in-depth discussions of such topics as free radicals, cancer, mercury toxicity, heart disease, inflammation, and many others. Highly recommended for the health professional or advanced student of nutrition.

Preventive Medicine Update
HealthComm, Inc.
5800 Soundview Drive
Gig Harbor, WA 98335
(800)-843-9660
PMU is a monthly service of HealthComm, Inc. Each month, subscribers receive a one-hour cassette featuring a discussion of the latest findings in nutrition by one of the country's most noted nutritional biochemists, Jeffrey Bland, Ph.D. Summary cards are included so subscribers can follow up on the studies discussed. The series also features monthly interviews with noted practitioners who offer clinical pearls and unique insights into how they use nutrition therapeutically. A sample tape is available for those interested in subscribing. Subscription includes one database search per year. Highly recommended.

ITS Services
3301 Alta Arden #3
Sacramento, CA 95825
(800) 422-9887
ITS Services isolates the latest studies on nutrition and puts them in abstract form. An excellent resource for nutritionists and health professionals who want to see summations of the latest research. They offer a monthly newsletter and a yearly compendium of abstracts. Indispensable.

The Quarterly Review of Natural Medicine
Natural Product Research Consultants, Inc.
600 First Avenue, Suite 205
Seattle, WA 98104
(206) 623-2520
Donald Brown, N.D. and his staff have done an excellent job supplying much-needed translations and reviews of recent studies in herbal medicine. Health professionals and students of herbal medicine will find it an invaluable resource for helping them understand what the latest findings mean and how to implement them in their practice.

Notes

1. "Americans Reducing Fat in Diet," Jane Brody, *New York Times*, March 8, 1994.

2. "Polyphenols and Bioflavonoids: The Medicines of Tomorrow: Part II," Brian E. Leibovitz, *Townsend Letter for Doctors*, May 1994, 436–39.

3. *Plant Flavonoids in Biology and Medicine*, vol. II, V. Cody, E. Middleton Jr., A. Beretz, eds., New York: Alan R. Liss, 1988.

4. "Iron Supplements May Raise Cancer Risk in the Elderly," *Geriatric Consultant*, March/April 1990; 6.

5. "Is Excess Iron Carcinogenic?" Peter Reizenstein, *Medical Oncology and Tumor Pharmacology*, 1990; 7 (1) :1–2.

6. "Role of Insulin Resistance in Human Disease," G. M. Reaven, *Diabetes*, 1988; 37; 1,595–1,607.

7. "Hyperinsulinemia, Sex, and the Risk of Atherosclerotic Cardiovascular Disease," M. Modan, et al, *Circulation*, 1991; 84; 1,165–75.

8. "Essential Fatty Acids and Dietary Endocrinology: A Hypothesis for Cardiovascular Treatment," Barry Sears, Ph.D., *Journal of Advancement in Medicine*, winter 1993; 6: 4, 211–24.

9. "Alteration of Cellular Fatty Acid Profile and the Production of Eicosonoids in Human Monocytes by GLA," Sally Pullman-Mooar, et al, *Arthritis and Rheumatism*, October 1990; 33 (10): 1,526–32.

10. *Journal of the National Cancer Institute*, G. A. Boissonneault, et al, 76:335–37, 1986.

11. *Nutrition and Cancer*, H. N. Englyst, et al, 4:50–58, 1982.

12. "Dietary Fat and Cancer Trends," M. G. Enig, et al, *Federal Proceedings*, 37:2,215–19, 1978.

13. *Lancet*, 1993; 341: 581.

14. "Modification of Membrane Lipid Composition and Mixed-Function Oxidases in Mouse Liver Microsomes by Dietary Trans Fatty Acids," M. G. Enig, 1984, Doctoral Dissertation, University of Maryland, College Park, MD.

15. "Effect of Dietary Trans Fatty Acids on High Density and Low Density Lipoprotein Cholesterol Levels in Healthy Subjects," R. P. Mensink, and M. B. Katan, *The New England Journal of Medicine* 323: 439–45.

16. "Dietary Factors and Breast Cancer Risk in Denmark," M. Ewertz, and C. Gill, *International Journal of Cancer* 46: 779–84.

17. *Trans Fatty Acids in the Food Supply: A Comprehensive Report Covering 60 Years of Research*, Mary Enig, Ph.D., Enig Associates, Silver Spring, MD, 1993.

18. "Dietary Factors in Hormone-Dependent Cancers," K. K. Carroll, in *Current Concepts in Nutrition*, vol. 6., *Nutrition and Cancer*, New York: John Wiley and Sons, 1977, 25–40.

19. "Diet and Breast Cancer: The Possible Connection with Sugar Consumption," S. Seely and D. F. Horrobin, *Medical Hypotheses*, 11 (3): 319–27, 1983.

20. "Dietary Sugar Intake in the Etiology of Biliary Tract Cancer," Clara J. Moerman, et al, *International Journal of Epidemiology*, 1993; 22: 207–14.

21. "Evidence that Glucose Ingestion Inhibits Net Renal Tubular Reabsorption of Calcium and Magnesium," J. Lemann, *Journal of Laboratory and Clinical Medicine*, 70: 236–45.

22. "Dietary Fat and Dietary Sugar in Relation to Ischemic Heart Disease and Diabetes," J. Yudkin, *Lancet*, 1964, 2:4.

23. "Diets High in Glucose or Sucrose and Young Women," J. Kelsay, et al, *American Journal of Clinical Nutrition*, 1974, 27: 926–36.

24. "Effects of Dietary Sugars on Metabolic Risk Factors Associated with Heart Disease," S. Reiser, *Nutritional Health*, 1985, 3:203–16.

25. "Carbohydrates and Blood Pressure," R. Hodges and T. Rebello, *Annals of Internal Medicine*, 1983, 98: 838–41.

26. "The Effect of Dietary Sucrose on Blood Lipids, Serum Insulin, Platelet Adhesiveness and Body Weight in Human Volunteers," S. Scanto and John Yudkin, *Postgraduate Medical Journal*, 1969, 45: 602–7.

27. "Role of Sugars in Human Neutrophilic Phagocytosis," A. Sanchez, et al, *American Journal of Clinical Nutrition*, November 1973, 1,180–84.

28. "Sucrose, Neutrophilic Phagocytosis and Resistance to Disease," W. Ringsdorf, E. Cheraskin, and R. Ramsay, *Dental Survey*, 52, 12: 46–48.

29. "Effect of Copper Deficiency on Metabolism and Mortality in Rats Fed Sucrose or Starch Diets," M. Fields, et. al., *Journal of Nutrition*, 1983, 113: 1,335–45.

30. *Diabetes, Coronary Thrombosis and the Saccharine Disease*, T. Cleave and G. Campbell, Bristol, England: John Wright and Sons, 1960.

31. "Effects of High Dietary Sugar," J. Yudkin, et al, *British Journal of Medicine*, November 22, 1980, 281: 139.

32. "Placebo Controlled Blind Study of Dietary Manipulation Therapy in Rheumatoid Arthritis," L. Darlington, Ramsay and Mansfield, *Lancet*, February 6, 1986, 236–38.

33. "Food Allergies and Migraine," E. Grand, *Lancet*, 1979, 1:955–59.

34. "The Sweet Road to Gallstones," K. Heaton, *British Medical Journal*, April 14, 1984, 228: 1,103–4.

35. "Nutrient Intake, Adiposity and Diabetes," H. Keen, et al, *British Medical Journal*, 1974, 655–58.

36. *The Saccharine Disease*, T. Cleave, New Canaan, CT: Keats Publishing, 1974.

37. *Sweet and Dangerous*, J. Yudkin, New York: Bantam Books, 1974.

38. *Sugar Blues*, W. Duffy, New York: Warner Books, 1975.

39. *Lick the Sugar Habit*, Nancy Appleton, Garden City, NY: Avery Publishing Group, 1988.

40. *Cancer Letters*, 68: 231–36, 1993.

41. *British Journal of Cancer*, 67: 424–29, 1993.

42. "Dietary Antioxidant Flavonoids and Risk of Coronary Artery Disease: The Zutphen Elderly Study," M. G. L. Hertog, E. J. M. Feskens, et al, *Lancet*, 342: 1,007–11, 1993.

43. "Essential Fatty Acids and Inflammation," B. Zurier, *Annals of Rheumatic Diseases*, 1991;50:745–46.

44. "Hand Handicap and Rheumatoid Arthritis in a Fish Eating Society (Faroe Islands)," L. Recht, et al, *Journal of Internal Medicine*, 1990; 227:49–55.

45. "Effects of Fish Oil Supplementation in Rheumatoid Arthritis," Hille Van Der Tempel, et al, *Annals of Rheumatic Diseases*, 1990; 49: 76–80.

46. "Vitamin E Status During Dietary Fish Oil Supplementation in Rheumatoid Arthritis," Jacob E. Tulleken, et al, *Arthritis and Rheumatism*, September 1990; 33 (9): 1,416–19.

47. "Dietary Fish Oil and Rheumatic Diseases," Geraldine McCarthy and Dermot Kenny, *Seminars in Arthritis and Rheumatism*, June 1992; 21 (6): 368–75.

48. "Severe Rheumatoid Arthritis: Current Options in Drug Therapy," M. Joel Kremer, M.D., *Geriatrics*, December 1990; 45 (12): 43–48.

49. "Long Term Supplementation with Omega 3 Fatty Acids II: Effect on Neutrophil and Monocyte Chemotaxis," E. B. Schmidt, et al, *Scandinavian Journal of Clinical Laboratory Investigation*, 1992; 52: 229–36.

50. "Effects of Manipulation of Dietary Fatty Acids on Clinical Manifestations of Rheumatoid Arthritis," J. L. Kremer, et al, *Lancet*, 1: 184–87, 1985.

51. "Therapeutic Activity of Oral Glucosamine Sulfate in Osteoarthritis: A Placebo Controlled Double-Blind Investigation," A. Drovanti, et al, *Clinical Therapy*, 1980; 3: 260–72.

52. "Decreased Incorporation of 14C-Glucosamine Relative to 3H-N-Acetyl Glucosamine in the Intestinal Mucosa of Patients with Inflammatory Bowel Disease," A. Burton, et al, *American Journal of Gastroeneterology*, 1983, 78 (1): 19–22.

53. "An Antioxidant a Day Keeps the Doctor in the Pink," Bruce Jancin, *Family Practice News*, March 1, 1994; 10.

54. *Chemical Sensitivity*: vol. II, *The Total Load*, Shari Rogers, 1994.

55. "Low Thyroxin Levels in Female Psychiatric Patients with Riboflavin Deficiency: Implications for Folate Dependent Methylation," I. R. Bell, et al, *ACTA Psychiatrica Scandinavia*, 1992; 85: 360–63.

56. "Human Obesity," *Contemporary Nutrition*, 1993, 18; 7,8: 1–4.

57. "Effect of Pyridoxine Supplementation on Recurrent Stone Formers," M. S. R. Murthy, et al, *International Journal of Clinical Pharmacology, Therapy and Toxicology*, 1982.

58. "Primary Oxalosis: Clinical and Biochemical Response to High-Dose Pyridoxine Therapy," E. J. Will and O. L. Bijvoet, *Metabolism* 28 (5): 542–48, 1979.

59. "Effects of Magnesium Hydroxide in Renal Stone Disease," G. Johansson, et al, *Journal of the American College of Nutrition* 1 (2) ; 1982.

60. "Nutritional Factors in Calcium Containing Kidney Stones with Particular Emphasis on Vitamin C," J. W. Piesse, *International Clinical Nutrition Reviews* 5 (3): 110–29, 1985.

61. "Effect of High Dose Vitamin C on Urinary Oxalate Levels," Theodore R. Wandzilak, et al, *Journal of Urology*, April 1994; 151: 834–37.

62. "Vitamin Deficiency and Mental Symptoms," M. W. P. Carney, *British Journal of Psychiatry*, 1990; 156:878–82.

63. "Reduced Activities of Thiamine Dependent Enzymes in the Brains and Peripheral Tissues of Patients with Alzheimer's Disease," G. Gibson, et al, *Archives of Neurology* 45:836–40, 1988.

64. "A Trial of Thiamine in Alzheimer's Disease," K. A. Nolan, et al, *Archives of Neurology*, January 1991;48:81–83.

65. "Thiamine Deficiency," Gregory L. Brotzman, M.D., *Journal of the American Board of Family Practice*, May/June 1992; 5 (3): 323–25.

66. "Diabetic Polyneuropathy and Vitamin B1," V. Frydl and H. Zavodska, *Medwelt*, 1989; 40: 1,484–86.

67. "The Effect of a Nutritional Supplement On Premenstrual Symptomatology in Women with Premenstrual Syndrome: A Double Blind Longitudinal Study," R. S. London, et al, *Journal of the American College of Nutrition*, 1991; 10(5):494–99.

68. "Nutritional Approach to Cancer Prevention with Emphasis on Vitamins, Antioxidants and Carotenoids," John H. Weisburger, *American Journal of Clinical Nutrition*, 1991;53:226S–237S.

69. "Increased Plasma Lipid Peroxidation in Riboflavin-Deficient Malaria-Infected Children," S. Bhabani Das, et al, *American Journal of Clinical Nutrition*, 1990; 51:859–63.

70. "Riboflavin Excretion in Normal and Diabetic Rats," Alluru S. Reddi, et al, *International Journal of Vitamin and Nutrition Research*, 1990; 60: 252–54.

71. "Niacin—The Long and the Short of It," Mary J. Malloy, M.D., et al, *The Western Journal of Medicine*, October 1991;155:426.

72. "The Effects of Nicotinic Acid on Serum Cholesterol Concentrations of High Density Lipoprotein Subfractions HDL2 and HDL3 and Hyperproteinemia," G. Wahlberg, et al, *Journal of Internal Medicine*, 1990; 228: 151–57.

73. "Normalization of Composition of Very Low Density Lipoproteins In Hypertriglyceridemia by Nicotinic Acid," Per Tornvall, et al, *Atherosclerosis*, 1990; 84: 219–27.

74 "How Safe Is Niacin for Cholesterol Reduction?" *Patient Care*, December 15, 1990; 123.

75. "Management of the Patient with a Low HDL-Cholesterol," R. F. Leighton, M.D., *Clinical Cardiology*, August 1990; 13:521–32.

76. "Cholesterol: Low-Dose Niacin Well-Tolerated," *Modern Medicine*, January 1990; 58; 31.

77. "Marked Benefit with Sustained-Release Niacin Therapy in Patients with 'Isolated' Very Low Levels of High-Density Lipoprotein Cholesterol and Coronary Artery Disease," Carl J. Lavie, M.D., et al, *The American Journal of Cardiology*, April 15, 1992; 69: 1,083–85.

78. "Atherosclerosis: The Importance of HDL Cholesterol and Prostacyclin: A Role for Niacin Therapy," M. H. Luria, *Medical Hypothesis*, 1990; 32: 21–28.

79. "Nicotinic Acid as Therapy for Dyslipidemia in Non-Insulin Dependent Diabetes Mellitus," Abhimanyu Garg, M.D., and M. Scott Grundy, M.D., Ph.D., *JAMA*, August 8, 1990; 264(6): 723–26.

80. "Niacin-Induced Diabetes," Richard A. Rubin, M.D., *Cortlandt Forum*, March 1992; 124/49–17.

81. "Niacin-Induced Hepatitis: A Potential Side Effect with Low-Dose Time-Released Niacin," Jeff A. Etchason, M.D., et al, *Mayo Clinic Proceedings*, 1991; 66: 23–28.

82. "Rechallenge with Crystalline Niacin After Drug-Induced Hepatitis from Sustained Release Niacin," Yaakov Henkin, M.D., et al, *JAMA*, July 11, 1990; 264 (2): 241–43.

83. "Acute Hepatic Failure Associated with the Use of Low-Dose Sustained Release Niacin," N. Howard Hodis, M.D., *JAMA*, July 11, 1990; 264: 2; 181.

84. "Vitamin B3 in the Treatment of Diabetes Mellitus: Case Reports and Review of the Literature," John P. Cleary, M.D., *Journal of Nutritional Medicine*, 1990; 1:217–25.

85. "Dietary Intakes and Plasma Concentrations of Folate in Healthy Adolescents," W. A. Daniel, et al, *American Journal of Clinical Nutrition*, 28: 363–70.

86. "Plasma Folate Adequacy as Determined by Homocysteine Levels," Charles A. Lewis, M.D., M.P.H., et al, *Beyond Deficiency: New Views on the Function and Health Effects of Vitamins*, New York Academy of Sciences, February 9–12.

87. "Pantethine: A Physiological Lipomodulating Agent, in the Treatment of Hyperlipidemia," G. C. Maggi, C. Donati, G. Criscuoli, *Curr. Ther. Res.*, 32: 380, 1982.

88. "Effect of Pantethine on Lipids, Lipoproteins and Apolipoproteins in Man," P. Avogaro, Bon G. Bittolo, M. Fusello, *Curr. Ther. Res.*, 33: 488, 1983.

89. "Controlled Evaluation of Pantethine, a Natural Hypolipidemic Compound, in Patients with Different Forms of Hyperlipoproteinemia," A. Gaddi, et al, *Atherosclerosis*, 50: 73, 1984.

90. "Effects of Supplemental Pantothenic Acid on Wound Healing: Experimental Study in Rabbit," Marc Aprahamian, et al, *American Journal of Clinical Nutrition* 41:March 1985, 578–89.

91. *Nutrition Against Disease*, Roger Williams, New York: Pitman Publishing, 1971, 126.

92. "Association of Vitamin B-6 Status with Parameters of Immune Function in Early HIV-1 Infection," Marianna K. Bum, et al, *Journal of Acquired Immunodeficiency Syndromes*, 1991; 4: 1,122–32.

93. "Relation of Short-Term Pyridoxine Hydrochloride Supplementation to Plasma Vitamin B-6 Vitamers and Amino Acid Concentrations in Young Women," Soon Ah Kang-Yoon and Avanelle Kirkey, *American Journal of Clinical Nutrition*, 1992; 55: 865–72.

94. "Acquired Atherosclerosis: Theories of Causation, Novel Therapies," Joseph G. Hattersley, M.A., *Journal of Orthomolecular Medicine*, 1991;6(2):83–98.

95. "Nutrition and Candidiasis," Leo Galland, M.D., *Journal of Orthomolecular Psychiatry*, 14:50–60, 1985.

96. "A Prospective Study of Plasma Homocysteine and Risk of Myocardial Infarction in U.S. Physicians," Meir J. Stamfer, M.D., et al, *JAMA*, August 19, 1992; 268 (7): 877–81.

97. "Vitamin B_6 Curbs Severe Nausea, Emesis in Gravida," *Family Practice News*, June 1–14, 1991:10.

98. "Nutrition and Candida Albicans," Leo D. Galland, M.D., *1986: A Year in Nutritional Medicine*, Keats Publishing, 1986:10–12.

99. "Diet and Hyperoxaluria and the Syndrome of Idiopathic Calcium Oxalate Urolithiasis," Lynwood H. Smith, M.D., *American Journal of Kidney Diseases*, April 1991;17(4):370–75.

100. "Electrophysiological Effects of Fenfluramine or Combined Vitamin B_6 and Magnesium on Children with Autistic Behavior," J. Martineau, et al, *Developmental Medicine and Child Neurology*, 1989; 31: 721–27.

101. "Effects of Pharmacologic Doses of B_6 on Carpal Tunnel Syndrome, Electroencephalographic Results, and Pain," A. L. Bernstein and J. S. Dinesen, *Journal of the American College of Nutrition*, 12 (1), 73–76.

102. "Vitamin B_{12} Status in a Macrobiotic Community," Donald R. Miller, et al, *The American Journal of Clinical Nutrition*, 1991; 53: 524–29.

103. "Myths About Vitamin B-12 Deficiency," Edward Fine, M.D., et al, *Southern Medical Journal*, December 1991; 1,474–81.

104. "Vitamin B-12 Injections," *American Family Physician*, February 1992;829–30.

105. "Cerebral Manifestations of Vitamin B_{12} Deficiency," Damien Downing, M.B., B.S., *Journal of Nutritional Medicine*, 1991; 2, 89–90.

106. "Subtle and Atypical Deficiency States," Ralph Carmel, M.D., *American Journal of Hematology*, 1990; 34: 108–14.

107. "Oral Cobalamin for Pernicious Anemia: Medicine's Best Kept Secret," Frank A. Lederle, M.D., *JAMA*, January 2, 1991; 265 (1): 94–95.

108. "Oral Cobalamin for Treatment of Pernicious Anemia?" John N. Hathcock, Ph.D., and Gloria J. Troendie, M.D., *JAMA*, January 2, 1991; 265 (1): 96–97.

109. "Orthostatic Hypotension Induced by Vitamin B_{12} Deficiency," A. Lossos, M.D., and Z. Argov, M.D., *Journal of the American Geriatric Society*, 1991;39:601–3. /56 1991

110. "Neurologic Signs of B_{12} Deficiency," Edward J. Fine, M.D., *Emergency Medicine*, July 15, 1992; 198–201.

111. "Molecular Basis for the Deficiency in Humans of Gluconolactone Oxidase, a Key Enzyme for Ascorbic Acid Biosynthesis," Morimitsu Nishikimi and Yagi Kunio, *The American Journal of Clinical Nutrition*, 1991;54:1,203S–1,208S.

112. "The New Scoop on Vitamins," Janice M. Horowitz, et al, *Time*, April 6, 1992; 54–59.

113. "Increased RDA for Vitamin C for Smokers May Still Be Too Low," *Family Practice News*, August 1–14, 1990; 20 (15): 29.

114. "Immunocompetence and Oxidant Defense During Ascorbate Depletion of Healthy Men," Robert A. Jacob, et al, *The American Journal of Clinical Nutrition*, 1991; 54: 1,302S–1,309S.

115. "Antihistamine Effects and Complications of Supplemental Vitamin C," Carol S. Johnston, Ph.D., R.D, et al, *Journal of the American Dietetic Association*, August 1992; 92 (8): 988–89.

116. "Radiation-Induced Neoplastic Formation of C3H102 1/2 Cells Suppressed by Ascorbic Acid," M. Yasukawa, et al, *Radiation Research*, 1989; 120: 456–67.

117. "Ascorbic Acid Metabolism in Protection Against Free Radicals: A Radiation Model," Richard C. Rose, *Biochemical and Biophysical Research Communications*, June 15, 1990; 169 (2): 430–36.

118. "Ascorbic Acid: Biological Functions and Relation to Cancer," Donald Earl Henson, et al, *Journal of the National Cancer Institute*, April 17, 1991;83(8):547–50.

119. "Vitamin C Levels in Patients with Familial Adenomatous Polyposis," A.D. Spigelman, et al, *British Journal of Surgery*, May 1990; 77 (5): 508–9.

120. "A Major Symposium on Vitamin C Sponsored by the National Cancer Institute," Morton A. Klein, Linus Pauling Institute of Science and Medicine,December 1990: 7.

121. "Vitamin C and Reduced Mortality," Gladys Block, *Epidemiology*, May 1992; 3(3): 189–91.

122. "Glutathione Blood Levels and Other Oxidant Defense Indexes in Men Fed Diets Low in Vitamin C," S. Henning, et al, *Journal of Nutrition*, 1991; 121: 169–75.

123. "Vitamin C and Cancer Prevention: The Epidemiologic Evidence," Gladys Block, *American Journal of Clinical Nutrition*, 1991;53: 2,701–282S.

124. "Dietary Factors and the Risk of Breast Cancer: Combined Analysis of Twelve Case-Controlled Studies," Geoffrey R. Howe, et al, *Journal of the National Cancer Institute*, 1990; 82: 561–69.

125. "Breast Cancer Rise: Due to Dietary Fat?" J. Raloff, *Science News*, April 21, 1990; 245.

126. "Direct Observation of a Free Radical Interaction Between Vitamin E and Vitamin C," J. E. Packer, T. F. Slater, and R. L. Wilson, *Nature*, 1979; 278:737–38.

127. "Antioxidant and Coantioxidant Activity of Vitamin C," T. Doba, G. W. Burton, and K. U. Ingold, *Biochem. Biophys. Acta.*, 1985; 835: 298–303.

128. "Antioxidants in Relation to Lipid Peroxidation," E. Niki, *Chem. Phys. Lipids*, 1987; 44: 227–53.

129. "Effect of Vitamin C on Transient Increase of Bronchoresponsiveness in Conditions Affecting the Upper Respiratory Airways," C. Bucca, et al, *Beyond Deficiency: New Views on the Function and Health Effects of Vitamins*, New York Academy of Sciences, February 9–12, 1992, Abstract 16.

130. "Vitamin C in the Treatment of Acquired Immune Deficiency Syndrome (AIDS)," R. Cathcart, M.D., *Medical Hypotheses* 14 (4): 423–32, 1984.

131. "AIDS: Remissions Using Nutrient Therapies and Megadose Intravenous Ascorbate," I. Brighthope, *International Clinical Nutrition Reviews*, 7 (2): 52–76, 1987.

132. "Vitamin C Reported to Cut Glycosylation," *Medical Tribune*, February 27, 1992.

133. "Effect of Vitamin C on Glycosylation of Proteins," J. Sarah Davie, et al, *Diabetes*, February 1992;41:167–73.

134. "Effects of Dietary Antioxidants on LDL Oxidation in Non-Insulin Dependent Diabetics," R. Brazg, et al, *Clin. Res.*, 1992; 40: 103A.

135. *Clinical Guide to the Use of Vitamin C: The Clinical Experiences of Frederick R. Klenner, M.D.*, Lendon H. Smith, M.D., Life Sciences Press, Tacoma 1988.

136. "Ascorbic Acid and Carnitine Biosynthesis," Charles J. Rabouche, *American Journal of Clinical Nutrition*, 1991;54:1,147S–1,152S.

137. "Vitamin C: From Scurvy to Ideal Vitamin Balance," H. Labadie, *La Presse Medicale*, December 7, 1991;20(42):2,156–58.

138. "Ascorbic Acid Protects Lipids in Human Plasma and LDL Against Oxidative Damage," Balz Frei, *The American Journal of Clinical Nutrition*, 1991;541,113S–541,118S.

139. "Vitamin C Seemed to Help Prevent CAD," David A. Strickland, *Medical World News*, August 1991;11.

140. "Influence of Antioxidant Vitamins on LDL Oxidation," I. Jailal, M.D., *Beyond Deficiency: New Views on the Functions and Health Effects of Vitamins*, New York Academy of Sciences, February 9–12, 1992;21.

141. See note number 61.

142. "The Role of Beta Carotene in Cancer Chemoprevention," Alberto Manetta and Carols Fuchtner, M.D., *Drug Therapy*, July 1992: 55–60.

143. "Role of Nutrition in Cancer of the Oral Cavity," John P. Richie, Ph.D., *Journal of Applied Nutrition*, 1991;43(1):49–57.

144. "Vitamin A Levels in Children with Measles in Long Beach, California," Antonio Arrieta, M.D., et al, *Journal of Pediatrics*, July 1992; 121 (1): 75–78.

145. "Vitamin A Reduces Morbidity and Mortality in Measles," Max Klein and Gregory D. Hussey, Editorial, *South African Medical Journal*, July 21, 1990; 78 (56–57).

146. "Vitamin A Levels and the Severity of Measles," Thomas R. Frieden, M.D., M.P.H., et al, *American Journal of Diseases in Children*, February 1992;146:182–86.

147. "The Interaction Between Vitamin A Status and Measles Infection," Greg Hussey and Max Klein, M.D., *Beyond Deficiency*, New York Academy of Sciences, February 9–12, 1992/Abstract 17.

148. "A Randomized, Controlled Trial of Vitamin A in Children with Severe Measles," Gregory D. Hussey and Max Klein, M.D., *The New England Journal of Medicine*, July 19, 1990; 323 (3): 160–64.

149. "Effect of Vitamin A Supplementation on Plasma Progesterone and Estradiol Levels During Pregnancy," Meena Panth, et al, *International Journal of Vitamin and Nutrition Research*, 1991;61: 17–19.

150. "Biochemical, Morphological and Functional Aspects of Systemic and Local Vitamin A Deficiency in the Respiratory Tract," H. K. Biesalski, et al, *Beyond Deficiency*, New York Academy of Sciences, February 9–12, 1992; P-5.

151. "Beta Carotene and Vitamin A: Casting Separate Shadows?" Thomas E. Edes, M.D., *The Nutrition Report*, February 1992;10(2);9, 16.

152. "Vitamin A and Provitamin A Levels in Epithelial Cancers: A Preliminary Study," P. Girija Ramaswamy, et al, *Nutrition and Cancer*, 1990; 14 (3 & 4): 273–76.

153. "Gout and Vitamin A Intoxication: Is There a Connection?" Anthony R. Mawson and Gabriel I. Onor, *Seminars in Arthritis and Rheumatism*, April 1991;20(5):297–304.

154. "Decreased Beta Carotene Tissue Levels in Uterine Leiomyomas and Cancers of the Reproductive and Nonreproductive Organs," Prabhudas R. Palan, Ph.D., et al, *American Journal of Obstetrics and Gynecology*, December 1989; 161 (6); Part I, 1,649–52.

155. "Antioxidant Micronutrients and Cancer Prevention," Joanne F. Dorgan, M.P.H., Ph.D., and Arthur Schatskin, M.D., Dr. P.H. *Hematology/Oncology Clinics of North America*, February 1991;5(1)43–68.

156. "Beta Carotene May Detoxify Carcinogens," Dan Hurley, *Medical Tribune*, August 20, 1992; 24.

157. "Nutrition and Breast Cancer," David Kritchevsky, Ph.D., *Cancer*, September 15, 1990; 66 (6): 1,321–24.

158. "Premalignant Lesions: Role of Antioxidant Vitamins in Risk Reduction and Prevention of Malignant Transformation," Vishwa N. Singh and Suzanne K. Gaby, *American Journal of Clinical Nutrition*, 1991; 53: 386S–390S.

159. "Beta Carotene and Cancer," H. B. Stahelin, *British Journal of Clinical Practice*, December 1990;44(11):543–45.

160. "Supplements May Protect the Colon," D. Charles Bankhead, *Medical World News*, August 1991;37.

161. The Effects of Beta Carotene on the Immune System in Cancer," George S. Hughes, *The Nutrition Report*, January 1992;10(1):1–8.

162. "Factors Associated with Age-Related Macular Degeneration: An Analysis of Data from the First National Health and Nutrition Examination Survey," J. Goldberg, et al, *American Journal of Epidemiology*, 128 (4): 700–710, 1988.

163. "Retinal Degeneration in Monkeys Induced by Deficiencies of Vitamin E or Vitamin A," K. C. Hayes, *Invest. Opthalmol.*, 13 (7): 499–510, 1974.

164. "Plasma Concentrations of Carotenoids After Large Doses of B-Carotene," Roth Mathews and M. Micheline, *American Journal of Clinical Nutrition*, 1990; 52: 500–501.

165. "Dietary Synthetic Beta-Carotene or Dunaliella Bardawil and Hepatic Lipid Peroxidation," G. Levin, A. Ben-Amotz, Shoshana Mokady, *Journal of Optimal Nutrition* 2 (3): 143–50.

166. "Immobile, Sun-Deprived Elderly at Risk of Vitamin D Deficiency," *Geriatrics*, July 1991; 46(7):68.

167. "Effect of Vitamin D Supplementation on Wintertime and Overall Bone Loss in Healthy Postmenopausal Women," Bess Dawson-Hughes, M.D. et al, *Annals of Internal Medicine*, October 1, 1991;115(7):505–12.

168. "Vitamin D Status Among Patients with Fractured Neck of the Femur in Hong Kong," K. K. Pun, et al, *Bone*, 1990; 365–68.

169. "Vitamin D Deficiency in Elderly People," J. Chalmers, *British Medical Journal*, August 3, 1991; 303: 314–15.

170. "Intestinal Absorption of Cholecalciferol and 25-Hyroxycholecalciferol in Patients with Crohn's Disease and Intestinal Resection," Georges A. Leichtmann, et al, *American Journal of Clinical Nutrition*, 1991;54:548–52.

171. "Additive Risk Factors in Atherosclerosis," F. A. Kummerow, B. H. S. Cho, et al, *American Journal of Clinical Nutrition* 1976; 29: 579

172. "How Much Vitamin D Is Too Much?" *Medical World News*, January 13, 1975, 100–103.

173. "Vitamin D in the Treatment of Osteoporosis," Takno Fujita, *PSEBM*, 1992; 199:394–99.

174. *Sunlight*, Kime, Zane, M.D., World Health Publications, Penryn, CA, 1980.

175. "Sunlight, Vitamin D and Osteomalacia in the Elderly," H. M. Hodkinson, et al, *Lancet* 1973; 1:910

176. "Vitamin E Status of U.S. Children," Adrianne Bendich, Ph.D., *Journal of the American College of Nutrition*, 1992; 11: (4): 441–44.

177. "Pharmacologic Doses of Vitamin E Improve Insulin Action in Healthy Subjects and Non-Insulin Dependent Diabetic Patients," Guiseppe Paolisso, et al, *American Journal of Clinical Nutrition*, 1993;57:650–56.

178. "Magnesium Deficiency-Induced Cardiomyopathy: Protection of Vitamin E," Anthony M. Freedman, et al, *Biochemical and Biophysical Research Communications*, August 16, 1990; 170 (3): 1990.

179. "Supplementation of Humans with Vitamin E," Irene Simon-Schnass, *Journal of Nutrition*, 1991;121:2,005.

180. "Nutrition and High Altitude," Irene M. Simon-Schnass, *Journal of Nutrition*, 1992; 122: 778–81.

181. "Vitamin E and Cancer Prevention," Paul Knekt, et al, *The American Journal of Clinical Nutrition*, 1991;53:283S–286S.

182. "Vitamin Supplement Use and Reduced Risk of Oral and Pharyngeal Cancer," Gloria Gridley, et al, *American Journal of Epidemiology*, 1992; 135 (10): 1,083–92.

183. "Plasma Retinol, Beta Carotene and Vitamin E Levels in Relation to Future Risk of Preeclampsia," A. Jendryczko and M. Drozdz, *Zent. Bl. Gynakol.*, 1989; 111: 1,121–23.

184. "Vitamin E Suppresses Increased Lipid Peroxidation in Cigarette Smokers," Etsto Hoshino, et al, *Journal of Parenteral and Enteral Nutrition*, May/June 1990; 14 (3): 300–305.

185. "Lipid Soluble Antioxidants Preserve Rabbit Corneal Cell Function," Ora Lux-Neuwirth and Thomas J. Millar, *Current Eye Research*, 1990; 9 (2): 103–9.

186. "Vitamin E Moves on Stage in Cancer Prevention Studies," Kara Smigel, *Journal of the National Cancer Institute*, July 1, 1992; 84 (13): 996–97.

187. "The Importance of Vitamin E in Human Nutrition," June K. Lloyd, *ACTA Pediatr. Scand.*, 1990; 79: 6–11.

188. "Vitamin E Protects Nerve Cells from Amyloid B Protein Toxicity," Christian Behl, et al, *Biochemical and Biophysical Research Communications*, July 31, 1992; 186 (2): 944–50.

189. *Fats and Oils*, Udo Erasmus, Vancouver, B.C.: Alive Publishing, 1986.

190. "Vitamin K and Human Nutrition," J.W. Suttie, Ph.D., *Journal of the American Dietetic Association*, May 1992; 92 (5): 585–90.

191. "Effects on Blood Pressure of Calcium Supplements in Women," N. Johnson, et al, *American Journal of Clinical Nutrition*, 42: 12–17, 1985.

192. "Blood Pressure Response to Oral Calcium in Persons with Mild to Moderate Hypertension," D. McCarron and C. Morris, *Annals of Internal Medicine*, 103: 825–31, 1985.

193. "Calcium and Colon Cancer: A Review," A. Sorenson, et al, *Nutrition and Cancer*, 11: 825–31, 1985.

194. "Effect of Added Dietary Cancer on Colonic Epithelial Cell Proliferation in Subjects at High Risk for Familial Colonic Cancer," M. Lipkin and H. Newmark, *The New England Journal of Medicine*, 313: 1,381–84, 1985.

195. "Magnesium Replacement Therapy," Joseph R. Dipalma, M.D., *AFP Journal*, July 1990; 173–76.

196. "Hypomagnesemia and Sudden Death in CHF Patients," Lawrence M. Prescott, Ph.D., *Practical Cardiology*, June 1990; 16 (6): 8.

197. "Prognostic Importance of Serum Magnesium Concentration in Patients with Congestive Heart Failure," Steven S. Gottlieb, M.D., et al, *Journal of the American College of Cardiology*, October 1990; 16 (4): 827–31.

198. "Magnesium for Restless Sleep," Burton Friedman, M.D., Cortlandt *Forum*, February 1992;121:48–10.

199. "Justification for Intravenous Magnesium Therapy in Acute Myocardial Infarction," H. S. Rasmussen, *Magnesium Research*, 1988; 1: 59–73.

200. "Magnesium for Suspected MI," Jacob E. Teitelbaum, M.D., *Cortlandt Forum*, March 1990.

201. "Intravenous Magnesium Sulfate in Suspected Acuts Myocardial Infarction: Results of the Second Leicester Intravenous Magnesium Intervention Trial (LIMIT-2)," Kent L. Woods, et al, *Lancet*, June 27, 1992; 339:1, 553–58.

202. "Magnesium and Acute Myocardial Infarction" (International Study of Infarct Survival Four), Mildred S. Seelig, M.D., *American Journal of Cardiology*, 1991, 1,221–22.

203. "Magnesium Said to Cut Post-MI Deaths," *Medical World News*, March 1992;16.

204. "The Role of Magnesium in Cardiac Arrhythmias," Peter K. Keller and Ronald S. Aronson, *Progress in Cardiovascular Diseases*, May/June 1990;32(6):433–448.

205. "Possible Use of Magnesium in the Clinical Treatment of Cardiac Arrhythmias," D. H. Antoni, *Magnesium Research*, 1988;1: 104 (10th Honheim Magnesium Symposium).

206. "Magnesium Deficiency in Coronary Artery Disease and Cardiac Arrhythmias," A. Sjogren, et al, *Journal of Internal Medicine*, 1989; 229: 213–22.

207. "Effect of Dietary Magnesium on Development of Atherosclerosis in Cholesterol-Fed Rabbits," Yasuyoshi Ouchi, et al, *Atherosclerosis*, September/October 1990; 10: 732–37.

208. "Suppression of Ventricular Arrythmias by Magnesium," Dan Tzivoni, M.D., and Andre Keren, M.D., *The American Journal of Cardiology*, June 1, 1990;65: 1,397–99.

209. "Magnesium Deficiency and Peripheral Vascular Disease," J. M. H. Howard, D,Sc., F.A.C.N., *Journal of Nutritional Medicine*, 1990; 1: 39–49.

210. "Renal Excretion of Lactate and Magnesium in Mitral Valve Prolapse," L. Cohen, et al, *Magnesium Research*, 1988; 1: 75–78.

211. "Stress and Magnesium Metabolism in Coronary Artery Disease," R. Smetena, et al, *Magnesium Bulletin*, 1991;13(4):125–27.

212. "Introduction: Magnesium—Coming of Age," David P. Lauler, M.D., *The American Journal of Cardiology*, April 18, 1989;1G–3G.

213. "Effects of Magnesium Supplementation on Strength Training in Humans," Lorraine R. Brilla, Ph.D., and Timothy F. Haley, B.S., R.N., *Journal of the American College of Nutrition*, 1992; 11 (3): 326–29.

214. "Magnesium and Insulin-Dependent Diabetes Mellitus," Abdelaziz Elamin and Torsten Tuvemo, *Diabetes Research and Clinical Practice*, 190; 10:203–9.

215. "Magnesium and Glucose Homeostasis," G. Paolisso, et al,. *Diabetologia*, 1990; 33:501–14.

216. "The Role of Magnesium Deficiency in Insulin Resistance: An In Vitro Study," Rastislav Dzurik, et al, *Journal of Hypertension*, 1991; 9 (Supplement 6): S312–S313.

217. "Association of Hypomagnesemia with Diabetic Retinopathy," A. Hatwal, et al, *ACTA Opthalmologica*, 1989; 67:714–16.

218. "Hypomagnesemia in Type II Diabetes Mellitus is Not Corrected by Improvement of Long Term Metabolic Control," Schnack, et al, *Diabetologia*, 1992;35:77–79.

219. "Nutrition and Candida Albicans," Leo Galland, M.D., in J. Bland, ed., *1986: A Year in Nutritional Medicine*, New Canaan, CT: Keats Publishing, 1986.

220. "Magnesium Chloride in Acute Diseases," Raul Vergini, M.D., *Townsend Letter for Doctors*, May 1990; 286.

221. "Low Magnesium as a Cause of Leg Cramps," Marion Friedman, M.D., *Cortlandt Forum*, June 1990; 37:28.

222. "Effects of Magnesium Salts in Preventing Experimental Oxalate Urolithiasis in Rats," Yoshihide Ogawa, et al, *The Journal of Urology*, August 1990; 144: 385–89.

223. "Low Blood Mononuclear Cell Magnesium Content in Hypocalcemia and Normomagnesemic Patients," Elisabeth Ryzen, M.D., et al, *The Western Journal of Medicine*, November 1987; 147: 549–53.

224. "Disorders of Magnesium Metabolism," Alan C. Alfrey, in *The Kidney: Physiology and Pathophysiology*, second edition, ed. D. W. Seldin and Giebischg, New York: Raven Press, 1992; 2357–73.

225. "Magnesium and Diabetes," *Practical Diabetology*, March/April 1991;10(2):1–5.

226. "Magnesium Deficiency in Patients with Ischemic Heart Disease With and Without Acute Myocardial Infarction Uncovered by Intravenous Loading Test," H. S. Rasmussen, et al, *Archives of Internal Medicine*, 148, 329–32, 1988.

227. "Magnesium Deficiency in Hypertension Uncovered by Magnesium Load Retention," C. B. Seelig, *American Journal of Clinical Nutrition*, 8 (5):455, abstract 113, 1989.

228. "Magnesium Deficiency Diagnosed by Intravenous Loading Test," L. Gullestad, et al, *Scandinavian Journal of Clinical and Laboratory Investigation.*, 1992; 52: 245–53.

229. "Effect of Magnesium Citrate and Magnesium Oxide on the Crystallization of Calcium Salts in the Urine: Changes Produced by Food-Magnesium Interaction," J. Lindberg, et al, *Journal of Urology*, 1990; 143: 248–51.

230. "Dietary, Total Body and Intracellular Potassium-to-Sodium Ratios and Their Influence on Cancer," Birger Jansson, Ph.D., *Cancer Detection and Prevention*, 1990; 14 (5): 563–65.

231. "Organic Foods vs. Supermarket Foods: Element Levels," Bob L. Smith, *Journal of Applied Nutrition*, 1993; 45 (1): 35–39.

232. "Potassium Depletion Exacerbates Essential Hypertension," G. Gopal Krishna, M.D., and Shiv C. Kapoor, Ph.D., *Annals of Internal Medicine*, July 15, 1991;115(2):77–83.

233. "Potassium and Ventricular Arrhythmias," Phillip J. Podrid, M.D., *The American Journal of Cardiology*, March 6, 1990; 65: 33E–44E.

234. "Hematologic Effect of Supplementing Anemic Children with Vitamin A Alone and in Combination with Iron," Luis Mejia, Ph.D., and Francisco Chew, *American Journal of Clinical Nutrition*, 1988; 48: 595–600.

235. *American Journal of Clinical Nutrition*, 1990; 52: 813.

236. "Ferrous Sulfate Reduces Thyroxine Efficacy in Patients with Hypothyroidism," N. R. C. Campbell, et al, *Annals of Internal Medicine*, 1992; 117: 1,010–13.

237. *Iron and Your Heart*, Randlall B. Lauffer, Ph.D., New York: St. Martins Press, 1991.

238. "Dietary Effects on Breast Cancer," Richard G. Stevens, et al, *Lancet*, July 20, 1991;338:186–87.

239. "The Effect of Iron on Experimental Colorectal Carcinogenesis," R. L. Nelson, et al, *Anticancer Research*, 1989; 9: 1,477–82.

240. "Dietary Iron and Colorectal Cancer Risk," Richard L. Nelson, *Free Radical Biology and Medicine*, 1992;12:161–68.

241. "Iron Overload in Psychiatric Illness," Paul Cutler, M.D., *American Journal of Geriatrics*, January 1991; 148:147–48.

242. "Is Parkinson's a Progressive Sidcrosis of Substantia Nigra Resulting in Iron and Melanin Induced Neurodegeneration?" M. B. H. Youdim, et al, *ACTA Neurol. Scand.*, 1989; 126:47–54.

243. "Iron Oxidation by Casein," T. Emery, *Biochemical and Biophysical Research Communications*, February 14, 1992; 182 (3): 1,047–52.

244. Clinical Utility of Serum Tests for Iron Deficiency in Hospitalized Patients," Edward R. Burns, M.D., et al, *American Journal of Clinical Pathology*, February 1990; 93: 240–45.

245. "Iron Depletion in Coronary Disease," Randall B. Lauffer, Ph.D., *American Heart Journal*, June 1990; 199 (6): 1,448.

246. "CoEnzyme Q10, Iron and Vitamin B_6 in Genetically-Confirmed Alzheimer's Disease," Masaki Imagawa, et al, *Lancet*, September 12, 1992; 340:671.

247. "Serum Ferritin and Stomach Cancer Risk Among a Japanese Population," Suminori Akiba, M.D., et al, *Cancer*, 1991;67:1,707–12.

248. "Anemia and Rheumatoid Arthritis: The Role of Iron, Vitamin B_{12}, and Folic Acid Deficiency and Erythropoieten Responsiveness," G. Vreugdenhil, *Annals of Rheumatic Diseases*, 1990; 49: 93–98.

249. "Low-Normal Iron Levels in Children Said to Warrant Supplementation," *Family Practice News*, January 15, 1992;22(2):41.

250. "Iron, Free Radicals and Cancer," Peter Reizenstein, *Medical Oncology and Tumor Pharmacology*, 1991; 8 (4): 229–33.

251. "Heme Iron Relative to Total Dietary Intakes of Iron—A Review," M. K. Sweeten, G. C. Smith, H. R. Cross, *Journal of Food Quality* 9:263–75.

252. "Iron," V. F. Fairbanks and E. Butler, in *Modern Nutrition in Health and Disease*, seventh edition, M. E. Shils and V. R. Young, eds., Philadelphia: Lea and Febiger, 1988, 193–226.

253. "Zinc Deficiency Tied to Neurofirbrillary Tangles in Alzheimer's," *Family Practice News*, October 15–31, 1990;20 (20): 7.

254. "Esophageal Cancer and Diet—A Case Controlled Study," M. Prasad, et al, *Nutrition and Cancer*, 1992; 18: 85–93.

255. "The Physiologic Role of Zinc as an Antioxidant," Tammy M. Bray, William J. Bettger, et al, *Free Radical Biology in Medicine*, 1990; 8: 281–91.

256. "Effect of Diabetes Type and Treatment on Zinc Status in Diabetes Mellitus," Jerome Honnorat, et al, *Biological Trace Element Research*, 1992; 32: 311–16.

257. "Zinc and Insulin Sensitivity," Patrice Faure, et al, *Biological Trace Element Research*, 1992; 32:305–10.

258. "Zinc in the Treatment of Diabetic Patients," B. Winterberg, et al, *Trace Elements in Medicine*, 1989; 6 (4): 173–77.

259. "Zinc Studies on Wound Healing," Magnus S. Agren, *Linköping University Medical Dissertations, #320*, Linköping, Sweden, 1990.

260. "Zinc for the Promotion of Wound Healing," Ananda S. Prasad, M.D., Ph.D., *Consultant*, May 1990; 15.

261. Zinc Sulfate for Macular Degeneration," *Geriatric Consultant*, May/ June 1992; 23, 28.

262. "Zinc and Macular Degeneration," *Nutrition Reviews*, July 1990;40(7): 286–87.

263. "Rapid Improvement in Dermatitis After Zinc Supplementation in a Patient with Crohn' s Disease," Douglas C. Heimburger, M.D., et al, *The American Journal of Medicine*, January 1990; 88: 71–73.

264. "The Role of Zinc in Reproduction: Hormonal Mechanisms," Alain-Emile Favier, *Biological Trace Element Research*, 1992; 32: 363–82.

265. "Effects of a Long Term High Magnesium Intake on Metabolism of Zinc in Sprague Dawley Male Rats," P. Laurant, et al, *Trace Elements in Medicine*, 1991;8 (2): 70–73.

266. "Assessment of Zinc Status in Oral Supplementation in Anorexia Nervosa," Neil I. Ward, Ph.D., *Journal of Nutritional Medicine*, 1990;1:171–77.

267. "Zinc Deficiency as a Model for Developing Chemical Sensitivity," Sherry A. Rogers, M.D., et al, *International Clinical and Nutrition Review*, January 1990; 10 (1): 253–58.

268. "Zinc and Clinical Medicine," C. J. McClain, *Journal of the American College of Nutrition*, 1990;9(5):545.

269. "Copper Needs Surveyed," *Medical Tribune*, October 18, 1990; 14.

270. "Effect of Copper Deficiency on Metabolism and Mortality in Rats Fed Sucrose or Starch Diets," Meira Fields, et al, *Journal of Nutrition*, 1983;113:1,335–45;11.

271. "Direct Relationship Between the Body's Copper/Zinc Ratio, Ventricular Premature Beats and Sudden Coronary Death," J. C. Spencer, *American Journal of Clinical Nutrition*, 32:1,184–85, 1979.

272. "Re: Serum Copper and the Risk of Acute Myocardial Infarction: A Prospective Population Study in Men in Eastern Finland," Leslie M. Klevay, *American Journal of Epidemiology*, 1992; 135 (7): 832–34.

273. "Serum Magnesium, Copper, and Zinc Concentrations in Acute Myocardial Infarction," I. K. Tan, et al, *Journal of Clinical Laboratory Analysis*, 1992; 6: 324–28.

274. "Relation of Serum Zinc and Copper to Lipids and Lipoproteins: The Yi People Study," Jiang He, M.D., et al, *Journal of the American College of Nutrition*, 1992; 11 (1): 74–78.

275. "Effect of Molybdenum or Iron Induced Copper Deficiency on the Viability and Function of Neutrophils from Cattle," R. Boyne and J. R. Arthur, *Res. Vet. Science,* 41(3):417–19, 1986.

276. "Candida Albicans Dimorphism and Virulence: Role of Copper," V. J. Vaughn and E. D. Weinberg, *Mycopathologica* 64(1):39–42, 1978.

277. "Copper May Cut Cardiac Deaths," Lynn Payar, *Medical Tribune,* July 26, 1990.

278. "Zinc and Copper Metabolism in Patients with Senile Macular Degeneration," B. Z. Silverstone, et al, *Ann. Opthalmol.,* 17 (7): 419–22, 1985.

279. "Effect of Experimentally Induced Chronic Copper Toxicity on Retina," D. K. Gahlot and K. S. Ratnakar, *Indian Journal of Ophthalmology,* 29 (4) :351–53, 1981.

280. "Lack of Effects of Copper Gluconate Supplementation," W. B. Pratt, et al, *American Journal of Clinical Nutrition* 42(4):681–82, 1985.

281. "Manganese: An Essential Nutrient for Humans," Jeanne Freeland-Graves, Ph.D., R.D., *Nutrition Today,* November/December 1988; 13–19.

282. "Essential Trace Elements in Antioxidant Processes," Sheri Zidenberg-Cherr and Carl L. Keen, *Trace Elements, Micronutrients and Free Radicals,* 1992; 107–27.

283. "Antioxidant Mechanism of Mn (II) in Phospholipid Peroxidation," Yoshiko Tampo and Masonari Yonaha, *Free Radical Biology and Medicine,* 1992; 13: 115–20.

284. "Hypoglycemia Induced by Manganese," A. H. Rubenstien, et al, *Nature,* 194:188–89, 1962.

285. "Low Levels of Manganese in Bronchial Biopsies from Asthmatic Subjects," M. J. Campbell, et al, *Journal of Allergy and Clinical Immunology,* January 1991;89.

286. "Effects of Manganese and Other Divalent Cations on Progressive Motility of Human Sperm," O. Mangus, et al, *Archives of Andrology,* 1990; 24: 159–66.

287. "Review of Studies with Chromium Picolinate in Humans: Part I–Part II," Gary W. Evans, Ph.D., *The Nutrition Report,* October-November 1989; 7(10–11); 73 and 81.

288. "Has Chromium Been Overlooked as a Hypolipidemic Agent?" Robert G. Lefavi, Ph.D., *The Nutrition Report,* September 1991;9(9):65,72.

289. "Chromium, Glucose Tolerance and Diabetes," Richard A. Anderson, *Biological Trace Element Research,* 1992; 32: 19–24.

290. "Urinary Chromium Excretion and Insulinogenic Properties of Carbohydrates," Richard A. Anderson, et al, *American Journal of Clinical Nutrition,* 1990; 51:864–68.

291. "Effect of Chromium Supplementation on Serum High-Density Lipoprotein Cholesterol Levels in Men Taking Beta-Blockers: A Randomized, Controlled Trial," John R. Roeback, Ph.D., *Annals of Internal Medicine,* December 15, 1991;115(12):917–24.

292. "The Effect of Chromium Picolinate on Serum Cholesterol and Apolipoprotein Fractions in Human Subjects," Raymond Press, et al, *Western Journal of Medicine,* January 1990; 152 (1): 41–45.

293. "Lipid Lowering Effect of a Dietary Nicotinic Acid–Chromium III Complex in Male Athletes," R. Lefavi, et al, *FASEB Journal,* 1991/ *The Nutrition Report,* July 1991;53.

294. "Evidence for Glycation Hypothesis of Aging from the Food-Restricted Rodent Model," E. J. Masoro and M. S. Katz, *J. Gerontology*, 44:B20–B22, 1989.

295. "Efficacy of Chromium Supplements in Athletes: Emphasis on Anabolism," Robert G. Lefavi, et al, *International Journal of Sports Nutrition*, 1992; 2:111–22.

296. "Selenium in Urea: Culprit or Bystander?" Mario Bonomini, M.D., et al, *Nephron*, 1992; 60: 385–89.

297. "Human Selenium Status and Glutathione Peroxidase Activity in North West England," D. J. Pearson, et al, *European Journal of Clinical Nutrition*, 1990; 44:277–83.

298. "Selenium Status in Disease: The Role of Selenium as a Therapeutic Agent," V. W. Bunker, Ph.D., et al, *British Journal of Clinical Practice*, 1990; 44 (8): 401–4.

299. "Selenium in Forage Crops and Cancer Mortality in U.S. Counties," Larry C. Clark, M.P.H., Ph.D., *Archives of Environmental Health*, January/February 1991;46(1)37–42.

300. "Serum Selenium and Subsequent Risk of Cancer Among Finnish Men and Women," Paul Knekt, et al, *Journal of the National Cancer Institute*, 1990; 82: 864–68.

301. "Selenium in Serum as a Possible Parameter for Assessment of Breast Disease," Helena Ksrnjavi and Dubravka Beker, *Breast Cancer Research and Treatment*, 1990; 16:57–61.

302. "Blood Selenium Concentrations and Glutathione Peroxidase Activities in Patients with Breast Cancer and with Advanced Gastrointestinal Cancer," Z. Pawlowicz, et al, *Journal of Trace Elements, Electrolytes and Health and Disease*, 1991; 5 (4): 275–277.

303. "Cot Death and Selenium," John C. FitzHerbert, *New Zealand Medical Journal*, July 24, 1991; 321.

304. "Effect of Selenium and Vitamin E on The Development of Experimental Atherosclerosis in Rabbits," J. Wojcicki, et al, *Atherosclerosis*, 1991; 87:9–16.

305. "Selenium Elevates Mood," *The Nutrition Report*, January 1992;10(1):7

306. "Selenium Supplementation Improves Mood in a Double Blind Trial," David Benton and Richard Cook, *Psychopharmacology*, 1990; 102: 549–50.

307. "Acute Pancreatitis – 'A Free Radical Disease' Decrease of Lethality by Sodium Selenite Therapy," Bodo Kuklinski, et al, *Z. Gesamte Inn. Med. Jahrg.*, 1991;46:S.1–52.

308. "Reduced Selenium in Asthmatic Subjects in New Zealand," Amber Flatt, et al, *Thorax*, 1990; 45:95–99.

309. "Selenium and the Immune Response," Gerhard N. Schrauzer, D.Sc., *The Nutrition Report*, March 1992; 10 (3): 17, 24.

310. "Selenium and Glutathione Peroxidase Variations Induced by Polyunsaturated Fatty Acid Oral Supplementation in Humans," Giuseppe Bellisola, et al, *Clinica Chimica Acta*, 1992; 205:75–85.

311. "Effect of Dietary Methionine on the Biopotency of Selenite and Selenomethionine in Rat," R. A. Sunde, et al, *Journal of Nutrition* 1981; 111:76–86.

312. "Selenium Distribution in Blood Fractions of New Zealand Women Taking Organic or Inorganic Selenium," J. A. Butler, et al, *American Journal of Clinical Nutrition* 1991; 53: 748–54.

313. *Science News*, 142: 404, December 12, 1992.

314. "Studies on Capsiacin Inhibition of Chemically Induced Lipid Peroxidation in the Lung and Liver Tissue of the Rat," A. K. De and J. J. Ghosh, *Phytotherapy Research* 6: 34–37, 1992.

315. "Thyme Species as Cough Medicines," F. C. Czygan and R. Hansel, *Zeitshrift fur Phytother.*, 14(2): 104–10, 1993.

316. "Effect of Turmeric and Curcumin on BP-DNA Adducts," M. A. Mukundan, M. C. Chacko, et al, *Carcinogenesis*, 1993, 14: 493–96.

317. "Antioxidants for Health and Disease Prevention," Nagaratnam Das, *Journal of Optimal Nutrition*, 2 (4): 217–21.

318. "This Fat May Fight Cancer in Several Ways," J. Raloff, *Science News*, 145: 12, March 19, 1994, 182–83.

319. "Hypercholesterolemic and Antiatherosclerotic Effects of Garlic in Goats—An Experimental Study," P. L. Kaul and M. C. Prasad, *Indian Veterinary Journal*, December 1990; 67:1,112–15.

320. "Garlic and Cardiovascular Risk Factors," J. Grunwald, *British Journal of Pharmacology*, 1990; 28: 582–83.

321. "Garlic Supplement for Lowering Cholesterol," Jill Stein, *Practical Cardiology*, October 1990; 16 (10): 7.

322. "Garlic Has to Smell Bad to Do Some Good," *Family Practice News*, November 15, 1992; 22 (6): 31.

323. "Garlic May Confer a Wide Range of Health Benefits," Christine Kilgore, *Family Practice News*, October 1–14, 1990; 20 (19): 45.

324. "First World Congress on the Health Significance of Garlic and Garlic Constituents, August 28–30, 1990," Robert I. Lin, Ph.D., *Nutrition Report*, 1990; 1–48.

325. "Garlic: A Review of Its Relationship to Malignant Disease," Judith G. Dausch, Ph.D., R.D., and Daniel W. Nixon, M.D., *Preventive Medicine*, May 1990; 19 (3): 346–61.

326. "Anticandidal and Anticarcinogenic Potentials for Garlic," Padma P. Tadi, M.S., et al, *International Clinical Nutrition Review*, October 1990; 10 (4): 423–29.

327. "Garlic's Potential Role in Reducing Heart Disease," M. Fogarty, *British Journal of Clinical Practice*, March/April 1993; 47(2): 64–65.

328. "Garlic Supplementation and Lipoprotein Oxidation Susceptibility," Stacy Phelps and William S. Harris, *Lipids*, 1993; 28 (5): 475–77.

329. "Effects of Garlic Coated Tablets in Peripheral Arterial Occlusive Disease," H. Kiesewetter, et al, *Clinical Investigator*, 1993; 71: 383–86.

330. "Garlic and Its Significance for the Prevention of Cancer: A Critical Review," E. Dorant, et al, *British Journal of Cancer*, 1993; 67: 424–29.

331. "Enhancement of Natural Cell Killer Activity in AIDS with Garlic," T. H. Abdullah, et al, *Dtsch. Zschr. Onkol.*, 21:52–54.

332. "Ginger Rhizome: A New Source of Proteolytic Enzyme," E. H. Thompson, et al, *Journal of Food Science* 38 (4), 652–55, 1973.

333. "Long-Term Effect of Bifidobacteria and Neosugar on Precursor Lesions of Colonic Cancer in CF1 Mice," Malcolm Koo and A. Rao, Venketshwer, *Nutrition and Cancer*, 1991;16:249–57.

334. "Bifidobacteria and Their Role in Human Health," T. Mitsuoka, *Journal of Industrial Microbiology*, 6 (1900) 263–68.

335. "Management of Herpes Simplex with a Virostatic Bacterial Agent," D. J. Weekes, 1983 *E.E.N.T. Digest* 25.

336. "Inhibition of Gastric Acid Secretion Reduces Zinc Absorption in Man," G. C. Sturniolo, et al, *Journal of the American College of Nutrition*, 1991; 4: 372–75.

337. *The Ultimate Nutrient: Glutamine*, Judy Shabert and Nancy Erlich, New York: Avery, 1994.

338. "Effects of Nutritive Factors on Metabolic Processes Involving Bioactivation and Detoxification of Chemicals," F. P. Guengerich, *Annual Review of Nutrition*, 1984; 4: 207–31.

339. "The Physiologic Effect of Ultraviolet Radiation," H. Laurens, *JAMA* 11: 2,385, 1939.

340. *Nutrition: Concepts and Controversies*, Eva Hamilton, Eleanor Whitney, and Frances Sizer, New York: West Publishing Company, 1988, 246.

341. "The Chemical Nature of Royal Jelly," G. F. Townsend and C. C. Lucas, *Biochem. J.*, 1940; 34: 1,155–62.

342. *Comp. Biochem. Physiol.*, K. J. O'Conner and D. Baxter, 1985; 81: 755–60.

343. "A Potent Antibacterial Protein in Royal Jelly," S. Fujiwara, et al, *The Journal of Biological Chemistry*, 265; 19, July 5, 1990, 11,333–37.

344. *Journal of Bacteriology*, C. S. McClesky and R. M. Melampy, 1938; 36: 324.

345. "Activity of 10-Hydroxydecenoic Acid from Royal Jelly Against Experimental Leukemia and Ascitic Tumors," G. F. Townsend, J. F. Morgan, B. Hazlett, *Nature*, May 2, 1959, 183: 1,270–71.

346. "Vitamin C: Topical Skin Protector," Douglas Darr, Ph.D., *The Nutrition Report*, July 1992; 10 (7): 49–59, 56.

347. "Biological Functions in Relations to Cancer," D. E. Henson, et al, *Journal of the National Cancer Institute*, 1991; 83: 847–850.

348. "Vitamin C Eyed for Topical Use as a Skin Preserver: The Compound Appears to Ward Off Sun Damage," *Medical World News*, March 1991;12–13.

349. "Zinc Salt Effects on Granulocyte Zinc Concentrations and Chemotaxis in Acne Patients," B. Dreno, et al, *ACTA Derm. Venereol. (Stockh.)*, 1992; 72: 250–52.

350. "Effect of Dietary Antioxidants on Actinic Tumor Induction," H. S. Black, *Res. Comm. Chem. Path. Pharmacol.* 7: 783, 1974.

351. "Fibrin Microclot Formations in Patients with Acne," L. Juhlin, et al, *Acta Derm. Venerol.*, 1983, 63: 538–39.

352. *Nutrition Almanac*, Lavon J. Dunne, New York: McGraw Hill, 1990, 141.

353. "Hair Growth Promoting Activity of Tridax Procumbens," S. Saraf, et al, *Fitoterapia* 62 (6): 495–98, 1991.

354. "Nutrient Intakes and Dietary Patterns of Older Americans: A National Study," A. S. Ryan, et al, *Journal of Gerontology*, 47 (5): M145–M150, 1992.

355. "Vitamin Requirements of Elderly People: An Update," R. M. Russell and P. M. Suter, *American Journal of Clinical Nutrition*, 58: 4–14, 1993.

356. "Effect of Vitamin and Trace Element Supplementation on Immune Responses and Infection in Elderly Subjects," R. K. Chandra, *Lancet*, 1992; 340: 1,124–27.

357. "Serum Vitamin Concentrations of Vitamins A and E and Early Outcome After Ischemic Stroke," J. De Keyser, et al, *Lancet*, June 27, 1992; 339: 1,562–65.

358. "Dietary Status of the Elderly: Dietary Intake and Thiamine Pyrophosphate Response," H. K. Nichols and T. K. Basu, *Journal of the American College of Nutrition*, 1994; 13 (1); 57–61.

359. "Metabolic Evidence that Deficiencies of Vitamin B_{12}, Folate and Vitamin B_6 Occur More Commonly in Elderly People," E. Joosten, A. van den Berg, R. Riezler, et al, *American Journal of Clinical Nutrition*, 58: 468–76, 1993.

360. "Riboflavin Requirement of Healthy Elderly Humans and Its Relationship to Macronutrient Composition of the Diet," W. A. Boisvert, I. Mendoza, C. Castaneda, et al, *Journal of Nutrition* 123: 915–25, 1993.

361. "Vitamin B_6 Deficiency Impairs Interleukin II Production and Lymphocyte Proliferation in Elderly Adults," Simon Nikbin Meydani, et al, *The American Journal of Clinical Nutrition*, 1990;53:1,275–80.

362. "Vitamin B_{12} and Folate in Acute Geropsychiatric in Patients," Iris R. Bell, M.D., Ph.D., *The Nutrition Report*, January 1991;9(1):1,8.

363. "Protein Bound Cobalamin Absorption Declines in the Elderly," John D. Scarlett, et al, *American Journal of Hematology*, 1992; 39:79–83.

364. "Folate Deficient Neuropathy," T. E. Parry, et al, *ACTA Hematologica*, 1990; 84: 108.

365. "Vitamin E Supplementation Enhances Cell-Mediated Immunity in Healthy Elderly Subjects," Simin Nikbin Meyadaini, et al, *The American Journal of Clinical Nutrition*, 1990; 52:557–63.

366. "Protective Role of Dietary Vitamin E on Oxidative Stress in Aging," Mohsen Meydani, D.V.M., Ph.D., *Age*, 1992; 15: 89–93.

367. "Requirement and Supply of Vitamin C, E and Beta Carotene for Elderly Men and Women," H. Heseker and R. Schneider, *European Journal of Clinical Nutrition*, 1994, 48, 118–27.

368. "Intake of Vegetables, Fruits, Beta Carotene, Vitamin C and Vitamin Supplements and Cancer Incidence Among the Elderly: A Prospective Study," A. Shibata, et al, *British Journal of Cancer* 66: 673–79, 1992.

369. "Use of Magnesium in the Management of Dementias," J. Leslie Glick, *Medical Sciences Research*, 1990; 18: 831–33.

370. "High Stored Iron Levels Are Associated with Excess Risk of Myocardial Infarction in Eastern Finnish Men," J. T. Salonen, et al, *Circulation*, 1992; 86: 803–11.

371. "Nutrition Requirements of the Elderly," H. N. Munro, et al, *Annual Review of Nutrition* 7, (1987): 23–49.

372. "Evidence of Cellular Zinc Depletion in Hospitalized But Not Healthy Elderly Subjects," Helen F. Goode, et al, *Age and Aging*, 1991;20:345–48.

373. "Zinc Utake by Primate Retinal Pigment in Epithelium and Choriod," David A. Newsome, et al, *Current Eye Research*, 1992; 11 (3): 213–17.

374. "Therapeutic Role of Zinc in Disease States," S. Ananda Prasad, M.D., Ph.D., *Nutrition and the M.D.*, May 1991;17(5):1–2.

375. "Lymphocyte Response is Enhanced by Supplementation of Elderly Subjects with Selenium-Enriched Yeast," A. Peretz, et al, *American Journal of Clinical Nutrition* 1991; 53: 1,323–28.

376. "Ginkgo Biloba Extracts," U. Stein, *Lancet*, February 24, 1990;335: 475–76.

377. "A Double-Blind Placebo Controlled Study of Ginkgo Biloba Extract (Tanakan) in Elderly Outpatients with Mild to Moderate Memory Impairment," G. S. Rai, M.D., et al, *Current Medical Research and Opinion*, 1991; 12(6):350–55.

378. "Influence of Gingko Biloba on Cyclosporin A Induced Lipid Peroxidation in Human Liver Microsomes in Comparison to Vitamin A, Glutathione and N-Acetylcysteine," Barthe Signe Alexandra, et al, *Biochemical Pharmacology*, 1991;41(10):1,521–26.

379. "Ginkgo Biloba," J. Kleijnen and P. Knipschild, *Lancet*, November 7, 1992, 340 (8828): 1,136–39.

380. "Serum Antioxidant Vitamins and Risk of Cataract," P. Knekt, et al, *British Medical Journal*, 1992; 305: 1,392–94.

381. "Ocular Ascorbate Transport Metabolism," Richard Rose and Ann M. Dode, *Comp. Biochem. Physiol.*, 1991;108(2):273–85.

382. "Vitamin C Could Cut Cataract Risk," Tim Friend, *USA Today*, Life Section, September 18, 1990.

383. "Various Nutrients Studied for Cataract Prevention," *Geriatrics*, January 1991;46(1):24.

384. "Retinal Degeneration in Three-Month-Old Rhesus Monkey Infants Fed a Taurine-Free Human Formula," H. Imaki, et al, *J. Neurosci Res*, 18 (4): 602–14, 1987.

385. "Review: Antioxidant Protection of the Aging Macula," H. Gerster, *Age and Aging*, 1991;20:60.

386. "Taurine, Retinal Function," John B. Lombardini, *Brain Research Reviews*, 1991;16:151–69.

387. "Nutrition Almanac," Lavon J. Dunne, ed., New York: McGraw Hill, 1990, 147.

388. "Children and Passive Smoking: A Review," Anne Charlton, M.Ed., Ph.D., *The Journal of Family Practice*, March 1994; 38 (3): 267–77.

389. *Smoking: The Artificial Passion*, David Krogh, New York: W. H. Freeman, 1991.

390. "Glycemic Index of Foods," A. S. Truswell, *European Journal of Clinical Nutrition*, 46 (Supplement 2): S91–S101, 1992.

391. "Daily Magnesium Supplements Improve Glucose Handling in the Elderly," Giuseppe Paolisso, et al, *American Journal of Clinical Nutrition*, 1992; 55: 1,161–67.

392. "Garlic as a Natural Agent for the Treatment of Hypertension: A Preliminary Report," D. Foushee, et al, *Cytobios*, 1982, 34, 145–51.

393. "The Effects of Low Doses of N-3 Fatty Acid Supplementation on Blood Pressure in Hypertensive Subjects: A Randomized Controlled Trial," Kenneth Radack, M.D., et al, *Archives of Internal Medicine*, June 1991;151:1, 173–180.

394. "Fish Oil Supplements: The Use of Fish Oil Supplements to Reduce the Risk of Heart Disease Remains Controversial," Kathryn Bucci, Pharm.D., *American Pharmacy*, June 1992; NS32 (6): 48–50.

395. "Effects of a Fish Oil Supplement on Blood Pressure and Serum Lipids in Patients Treated for Coronary Artery Disease," Isabelle Bairati, M.D., Ph.D., et al, *Canadian Journal of Cardiology*, January/February, 1992; 8 (1): 41–46.

396. "Dietary Antioxidants and Blood Pressure," L. Cohen, et al, *American Journal of Clinical Nutrition*, 1990; 30th Annual Meeting; 512, Abstract 18.

397. "Ascorbic Acid Supplements and Blood Pressure—A Four Week Pilot Study," E. B. Feldman, *Beyond Deficiency: New Views on the Function and Health Effects of Vitamins*, New York Academy of Sciences, February 9–12, 1992;P-9.

398. "Is Calcium More Important than Sodium in the Pathogenesis of Essential Hypertension?" D. A. McCarron, *Hypertension*, 7 (4): 607–25, 1985.

399. "Increasing Calcium Lowers Blood Pressure: The Literature Reviewed," H. J. Henry, et al, *Journal of the American Dietetic Association*, 85: 182–85, 1985.

400. "Effect of Magnesium on Blood Pressure," T. Dyckner, et al, *British Medical Journal*, 286: 1,847–48, 1983.

401. "Potassium Depletion Exacerbates Essential Hypertension," G. Gopal Krishna, M.D., and Shiv C. Kapoor, Ph.D., *Annals of Internal Medicine*, July 15, 1991;115(2):77–83.

402. "Potassium Supplementation Lowers Blood Pressure and Increases Urinary Kallikrein in Essential Hypertensives," Gloria Valdes, et al, *Journal of Human Hypertension*, 1991;5:91–96.

403. "Potassium Supplementation for Hypertension: A Meta-Analysis," F. P. Cappuccio, et al, *Journal of Hypertension*, May 1991;9:465–73.

404. "Refractory Potassium Depletion," R. Whang, et al, *Archives of Internal Medicine*, 1992; 12: 40–45.

405. "Decrease of Taurine in Essential Hypertension," N. Kohashi, et al, *Japan Heart Journal*, January 1983.

406. "Potentiation of the Actions of Insulin by Taurine," W. G. Lampson, et al, *J. Physiol. Pharmacol.*, 61:457–62, 1983.

407. "Effect of CoQ10 on Structural Alterations in the Renal Membrane of Stroke-Prone Spontaneously Hypertensive Rats," H. Okamoto, et al, *Biochem. Med. Metabol. Biol.*, 1991; 45: 216–26.

408. *Biomedical and Clinical Aspects of Coenzyme Q*, K. Folkers and Y. Yamamura, eds., Amsterdam: Elsevier Science Publishers, 1984, 252–60.

409. "Urinary Salt Excretion and Stomach Cancer Mortality Among Four Japanese Populations," Shoichiro Tsugane, et al, *Cancer Causes and Control*, 1991;2:165–68.

410. "Diet and Stomach Cancer Incidence: A Case-Control Study in Turkey," Taner Demirer, M.D., et al, *Cancer*, May 15, 1990; 65 (10): 2,344–48.

411. "Is Reduction of Dietary Salt a Treatment for Hypertension?" Lawrence R. Krakoff, *American Journal of Public Health*, 1991;41–42.

412. "Dietary Prevention of Hypertension Emphasized," Rachelle Du Bain, *Medical Tribune*, June 11, 1992.

413. "The Rise and Fall of Ischemic Heart Disease," R. A. Stallones, *Scientific American* 243: 53–59, 1980.

414. "News," Circulation Research, 70: A1,081, 1992.

415. "Nutrition and Heart Disease Part I: Basic Aspects," Brian Leibovitz and Jennifer Mueller, *Journal of Optimal Nutrition* 2 (3): 151–72.

416. "Vitamin B$_6$ and Arteriosclerosis," F. Kuzuya, *Nagoya J. Med. Sci.* 1993; 55: 1–9.

417. *New England Journal of Medicine*, 1991; 324: 1,149–55.

418. *Journal of the American Medical Association*, 1992; 268: 877–81.

419. "Prevalence of Familial Hyperhomocysteinemia in Men with Premature Coronary Artery Disease," Jacques J. Genest, Jr., M.D., et al, *Arteriosclerosis and Thrombosis*, September/October 1991;11(5):1,129–36.

420. "Homocystenuria," Oebele F. Brouwer, M.D., and J. M. Visy, M.D., *Neurology*, June 1992; 42; 1,254.

421. "Hyperhomocysteinemia: An Independent Risk Factor for Vascular Disease," Robert Clarke, M.R.C.P.I., et al, *New England Journal of Medicine*, April 25, 1991;324(17):1991.

422. *American Journal of Clinical Nutrition*, 1993; 57: 175–81.

423. "Potential Role of Beta Carotene in the Prevention of Cardiovascular Disease," Helga Gerster, *International Journal of Vitamin and Nutrition Research*, 1991;61:277–91.

424. "Beta Carotene and Cardiovascular Disease," Charles H. Hennekens, M.D., et al, "Beyond Deficiency: New Views on the Function and Health Effects of Vitamins," *New York Academy of Sciences*, February 9–12, 1992:22.

425. "Inhibition of LDL Oxidation by Beta Carotene," Ishwarial Jialal, *Circulation*, Supplement II, October 1991; 84(4):II–449/Abstract 1789.

426. "Beta-Carotene Role as Protector Gauged," *Medical Tribune*, November 29, 1990; 2.

427. "Role of Vitamin E in Prevention the Oxidation of Low-Density Lipoprotein," Hermann Esterbauer, et al, *The American Journal of Clinical Nutrition*, 1991;53,314S–53,321S.

428. "Serum Ascorbic Acid and HDL Cholesterol in a Healthy, Elderly Japanese Population," Roichi Itoh, et al, *International Journal of Vitamin and Nutrition Research*, 1990;60:360–65.

429. "Effect of Vitamin C on HDL and Blood Pressure," P. F. Jacques, *Journal of the American College of Nutrition*, 1990; 9 (5): 554/Abstract 106.

430. "Vitamin C and Plasma Cholesterol," Harri Hemila, *Critical Reviews in Food Science and Nutrition*, 1992; 32 (1): 33–57.

431. "Vitamin C and Cardiovascular Disease: A Review," Joel A. Simon, M.D., M.P.H., *The American College of Nutrition*, 1992; 11 (2): 107–25.

432. A Prospective Study of Vitamin C and the Incidence of Coronary Heart Disease in Women," J. Manson, et al, *Circulation*, 1992; 85: 865.

433. "Vitamin C and Heart Disease," Joel A. Simon, *The Nutrition Report*, August 1992; 10 (8): 58, 64.

434. "Effect of Vitamin C on High Density Lipoprotein Cholesterol and Blood Pressure," Paul F. Jacques, Sc.D., *Journal of the American College of Nutrition*, 1992; 11 (2): 139–144.

435. "Protective Role of Ascorbic Acid Against Lipid Peroxidation and Myocardial Injury," S. Chakrabarty, et al, *Molecular and Cell Biochemistry*, 1992; 111: 41–47.

436. "How Vitamin C Can Prevent a Heart Attack and Stroke," *Linus Pauling Institute for Science and Medicine Newsletter*, March 1992; 3.

437. "Inverse Correlation Between Plasma Vitamin E and Mortality from Ischemic Heart Disease in Cross-Cultural Epidemiology," K. F. Gey, et al, *ACTA Cardiologica*, 1989; 44 (6): 493–94.

438. "Hypercholesterolemic Effect of Vitamin E on Cholesterol-Fed Rabbit," Chopaga Phonpanichresamee, et al, *International Journal of Vitamin and Mineral Research*, 1990; 60: 240–44.

439. "Plasma Antioxidants and Coronary Heart Disease: Vitamins C and E and Selenium," R. A. Riemersma, et al, *European Journal of Clinical Nutrition*, 1990; 44: 143–50.

440. "Inverse Correlation Between Vitamin E and Mortality from Ischemic Heart Disease in Cross Cultural Epidemiology," K. F. Gey, P. Puska, P. Jordan, and U. K. Moser, *American Journal of Clinical Nutrition*, 1991; 53:326S–334S.

441. "Effect of Dietary Supplementation with Alpha Tocopherol on Oxidative Modification of Low Density Lipoprotein," Ishwarlal Jialal and Scott M. Grundy, *Journal of Lipid Research*, 1992; 33: 899–906.

442. "Myocardial Tissue Concentrations of Magnesium and Potassium in Men Dying Suddenly from Ischemic Heart Disease," C. J. Johnson, *American Journal of Clinical Nutrition*, May, 1979, 32: 967–70.

443. "Physiologic and Nutritional Importance of Selenium," J. Neve, *Experientia*, 1991;47: 187–93.

444. "Selenium and the Antioxidant Defense System," Raymond J. Shamberger, Ph.D., *Journal of the Advancement in Medicine*, spring 1992; 5 (1): 7–19.

445. "Relation Between Serum Selenium Concentrations and Atherogenic Index in Japanese Adults," Yoji Deguchi and Akira Ogata, *Tohoku J. Exp. Med.*, 1991; 165: 247–51.

446. "Selenium Deficiency Inhibits Prostacyclin Release and Enhances Production of Platelet Activating Factor by Human Endothelial Cells," Gerhardt Hampel, et al, *Biochemica et Biophysica Acta*, 1989; 1006: 151–58.

447. *New England Journal of Medicine*, 1993; 328: 608.

448. "Ultraviolet Radiation and Cholesterol Metabolism," R. Altshul and I. H. Herman, Seventh Annual Meeting of the American Society for the Study of Atherosclerosis, *Circulation* 8: 438, 1953.

449. "Inhibition of Experimental Cholesterol Arteriosclerosis by Ultraviolet Radiation," R. Altshul, *New England Journal of Medicine* 249: 96, 1953.

450. "Therapeutic Action of Ultraviolet Irradiation in a Complex Treatment of Patients with Initial Cerebral Atherosclerosis," L. A. Kunitsina, et al, *Soviet Med.* 33: 89, 1970.

451. "Influence of Graduated Sunlight Baths on Patients with Coronary Atherosclerosis," V. A. Mikhailov, *Soviet Med.*, 29: 76, 1966.

452. "Preventive Activity of Ultraviolet Rays in the Presence of Experimental Atherosclerosis," A. I. Pertsovskij, et al, *Vop Kurort Fizioter* 36: 203, 1971.

453. "Effects of Continuous and Impulse Ultraviolet Radiation Therapy in Clinical Health Resort Treatment of Patients with Hypertension and

Chronic Coronary Insufficiency," A. L. Goldman, et al, *Vop Kurort Fizioter* 36 (5): 417, 1972.

454. "Antioxidants and Atherosclerosis," Bernhard Hennig and Michal Toborek, *Journal of Optimal Nutrition*, 2 (4): 213–16.

455. "Ascorbic Acid Protects Lipids in Human Plasma and Low-Density Lipoprotein Against Oxidative Damage," B. Frei, *American Journal of Clinical Nutrition*, 54:1,113S–1,118S, 1991.

456. "Effects of Dietary Magnesium Deficiency and Excess D3 on Swine Coronary Arteries," Mashahiro Eto, M.D., et al, *Journal of The American College of Nutrition*, 1990; (2): 155–63.

457. "Atherosclerosis," *American Family Physician* 1987; 36 (6): 250.

458. "Egg Consumption and High-Density Lipoprotein Cholesterol," P. Schnohr, et al, *Journal of Internal Medicine*, 1994; 235: 249–51.

459. "KyoGreen: A Powerhouse of Nutrients," E. W. Lau, *Explore* 1993; 4; 1: 3–5.

460. "Edible Plant Extracts Modulate Macrophage Activity and Bacterial Mutagenesis," B. H. S. Lau, E. W. Lau, T. Yamasaki, *International Clinical Nutrition Review*, July 1992; 12; 147–55.

461. "Effects of B-Carotene Repletion on B-Carotene Absorption, Lipid Peroxidation, and Neutrophil Superoxide Formation in Young Men," Sohrab Mobarhan, et al, *Nutrition and Cancer*, 1990; 14: 195–206.

462. "Peroxyl Radical Scavenging by B-Carotene in Lipid Bilayers," Todd A. Kennedy and Daniel C. Liebler, *The Journal of Biological Chemistry*, March 5, 1992; 267 (7): 4,658–63.

463. "Carotenoids as Cellular Antioxidants," Louise M. Canfield, et al, *Proceedings in the Society of Experimental Biology and Medicine*, 1992; 200: 260–65.

464. "Effect of B-Carotene on Lymphocyte Subpopulations in Elderly Humans: Evidence for a Dose-Response Relationship," Ronald R. Watson, et al, *The American Journal of Clinical Nutrition*, 1991;53:90–94.

465. "Magnesium Concentration in Brains from Multiple Sclerosis Patients," M. Yasui, et al, *ACTA Neurol. Scand.*, 1990; 81: 197–200.

466. "In Vitro Activation of Peripheral Mononuclear Cells by Zinc in HIV-Infected Patients and Healthy Controls," T. Harrer, et al, *Clinical and Experimental Immunology*, 1992; 89: 285–89.

467. "The Role of Zinc in Acquired Immunodeficiency Syndrome," M. Odeh, *Journal of Internal Medicine*, 1992; 231: 463–69.

468. "Study of Immune Function of Cancer Patients Influenced by Supplemental Zinc or Selenium-Zinc Combination," Mei Weide, et al, *Biological Trace Element Research*, 1991;28(1):11–20.

469. "Zinc Gluconate and the Common Cold: A Controlled Clinical Study," J. C. Godfrey, et al, *The Journal of International Medical Research*, June 1992; 20 (3): 234–46.

470. "Enhancement of the Immune Response by Selenium: Clinical Trials," Ann M. Peretz, et al, Arztl. Lab, 1990;36:299–304.

471. "Lymphocyte Response Is Enhanced by Supplementation of Elderly Subjects with Selenium-Enriched Yeast," Anne Peretz, et al, *American Journal of Clinical Nutrition*, 1991;53:1,823–28.

472. "Does the Selenium Level and Selenium-Dependent Enzyme Activity in Blood Plasma Correlate with Human Lymphocyte Subpopulations and Function?" Baj Zbigneiw, et al, *International Journal of Immunopathology and Pharmacology*, 1992; 5 (1): 13–21.

473. "Glutathione in Foods Listed in the National Cancer Institute's Health Habits and History Food Questionnaire," Dean P. Jones, et al, *Nutrition and Cancer*, 1992;17:57–75.

474. "Glutathione Deficiency and Human Immunodeficiency Virus Infection," Frank Stall, et al, *Lancet*, April 11, 1992;339:909–12.

475. "Glutathione Found to Suppress AIDS Virus in Human Cell Cultures," *Primary Care in Cancer*, May 1991;36.

476. "Glutathione Deficiency and Radiosensitivity in AIDS Patients," K. A. Vallis, *Lancet*, April 13, 1991;337:918–19.

477. "Immunomodulating Properties of Dimethylglycine in Humans," Charles D. Graber, et al, *Journal of Infectious Diseases*, January 1981, vol. 143, no. 1, 101–6.

478. "Recurrent Candidiasis: Adjuvant Immunotherapy with Different Formulations of Echinacin," E. Coeugniet and R. Kuhnast, *Therpiewoche* 36: 3,352–58, 1986.

479. "The Influence of Immune-Stimulating Effects of Echinacea Pupurea on the Course and Severity of Colds," D. Schoneberger, *Forum Immunologie*, 8: 2–12, 1992.

480. "Antiviral and Immunological Activity of Glycoproteins from Echinacea Purpurea," C. Bodinet and N. Beuscher, *Planta Medica* 57 (Supplement 2): A33, 1991.

481. "Flow-Cytometric Studies with Eleutherococcus Senticosus," B. Bohn, C. T. Nebe, C. Birr, *Arzneim-Forsch Drug Res.* 37: 1,193–96.

482. "Recent Progress in Immunopharmacology and Therapeutic Effects of Polysaccharides," G. Chihara, *Develop. Biol. Standard.* 1992; 77: 191–97.

483. "Oral Magnesium Successfully Relieves Premenstrual Mood Changes," Fabio Facchinetti, M.D., et al, *Obstetrics and Gynecology*, August 1991; 78 (2):177–81.

484. "PMS: Hints of a Link to Lunch Time and Zinc," K. A. Fackelmann, et al, *Science News*, October 27, 1990; 138: 263.

485. "Abnormal Essential Fatty Acid Levels in Plasma of Women with Premenstrual Syndrome," M. G. Brush, Ph.D., et al, *American Journal of Obstetrics and Gynecology*, 1984;150 (4): 363–66.

486. "The Importance of Magnesium in the Management of Primary Postmenopausal Osteoporosis," Guy E. Abraham, M.D., et al, *Journal of Nutritional Medicine*, 1991; 2: 165–78.

487. "Calcification in Atherosclerosis," A. Tanimura, D. H. McGregor, H. C. Anderson, *J. Exp. Pathol.*, 2: (4), 261–73, 1986.

488. "Recent Data on Magnesium and Osteoporosis," L. Cohen, *Magnesium Research*, 1988; 1:85–87.

489. "An Integrative Lifestyle: Nutrition Strategy for Lowering Osteoporosis Risk," Parris M. Kidd, Ph.D., *Townsend Letter for Doctors*, May 1992;400–405.

490. *Preventing and Reversing Osteoporosis: Everywoman's Essential Guide*, Alan Gaby, Rockland, CA: Prima Publishing, 1994, 29–36.

491. "Studies on the Role of Manganese in Bone Formation," R. M. Leach, et al, *Arch. Biochem. Biophys.*, 1969; 133: 22–28

492. "Reasons for Boning Up on Manganese," J. Raloff, *Science News*, 130 (27): 199, 1986.

493. "Serum Copper in Elderly Patients with Femoral Neck Fractures," D. Conlan, et al, *Age and Aging*, 1990; 19: 212–14.

494. "Vitamin K–Dependent Carboxylation Reactions," Ces Vermeer, *Beyond Deficiency: New Views on the Function and Health Effects of Vitamins*, Annual Meeting of the New York Academy of Sciences, February 9–12, 1992, Abstract 12.

495. *Lancet*, 1984; ii: 283.

496. *Annals of Internal Medicine*, 1989; 111: 1,001.

497. "Vitamin K–Dependent Carboxylation Reactions," Ces Vermeer, *Beyond Deficiency: New Views on the Function and Health Effects of Vitamins*, Annual Meeting of the New York Academy of Sciences, February 9–12, 1992, Abstract 12.

498. "A Possible Protective Effect of Nut Consumption on Risk of Coronary Heart Disease," G. E. Fraser, et al, *Archives of Internal Medicine*, 152: 1,416–23, 1992.

499. "A Double Blind Placebo Controlled Trial of Ascorbic Acid in Obesity," G. J. Naylor, et al, *Nutr. Health*, 1985, 425.

500. "Impaired Thermoregulation and Thyroid Function in Iron-Deficiency Anemia," John L. Beard, et al, *The American Journal of Clinical Nutrition*, 1990; 52: 813–19.

501. "Selenium's Role in Thyroid Found," Taryn Toro, *New Scientist*, January 26, 1991; 129:27.

502. "Effect of Selenium Supplementation in Hypothyroid Subjects of an Iodine or Selenium Deficient Area: The Possible Danger of Indiscriminate Supplementation of Iodine-Deficient Subjects with Selenium," B. Contempre, et al, *Journal of Clinical Endocrinology and Metabolism*, 1991;73(1):213–15.

503. "The Role of Selenium in Thyroid Hormone Action," Marla J. Berry and P. Reed Larsen, *Endocrine Reviews*, 1992; 13 (2): 207–20.

504. "Is Carnitine Essential in Children?" M. Giovannini, et al, *The Journal of International Medical Research*, 1991;88–102.

505. "Acetylcarnitine Is Low in Cord Blood and Cystic Fibrosis," J. D. Lloyd-Still, et al, *ACTA Pediatr. Scand.*, 1990;427–39.

506. "Influence of (-)-hydroxycitrate on Genetically and Experimentally Induced Obesity in the Rodent," A. C. Sullivan and J. Triscari, *American Journal of Clinical Nutrition*, 1977; 30: 767–76.

507. "A Non-Prescription Alternative in Weight Reduction Therapy," A. Conte, *American Journal of Bariatric Medicine*, summer 1993: 17–19.

Index

Jorge el curioso™
El puesto de limonada

Curious George®
Lemonade Stand

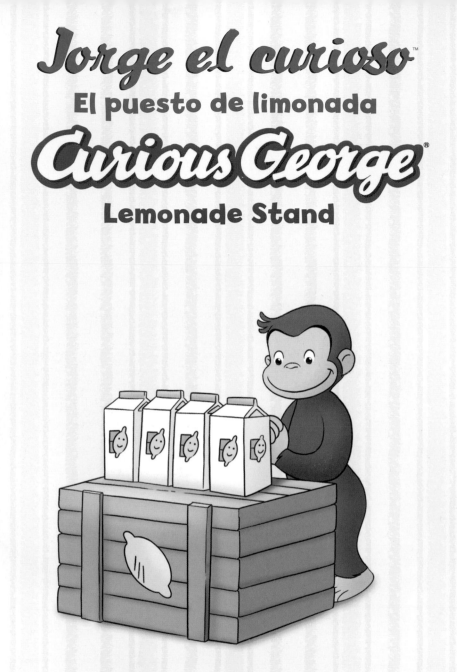

Adaptation by Erica Zappy Wainer
Based on the TV series teleplay "Curious George
Makes a Stand" written by Gentry Menzel

Adaptación de Erica Zappy Wainer
Basado en el programa de televisión "Curious George
Makes a Stand", escrito por Gentry Menzel
Traducido por Carlos E. Calvo

Houghton Mifflin Harcourt
Boston   New York

For information about permission to reproduce selections from this book, write to Permissions, Houghton Mifflin Harcourt Publishing Company, 215 Park Avenue South, New York, New York 10003.

ISBN: 978-0-544-65224-8 paper-over-board
ISBN: 978-0-544-65225-5 paperback

Design by Afsoon Razavi
Art adaptation by Rudy Obrero and Kaci Obrero

www.hmhco.com
Printed in Malaysia
TWP 10 9 8 7 6 5 4 3 2 1
4500570270

AGES	GRADES	GUIDED READING LEVEL	READING RECOVERY LEVEL	LEXILE ® LEVEL	SPANISH LEXILE ®
5–7	1	J	17	410L	480L